Nursing in contemporary society

£2

M

18/32

Nursing in contemporary society

Una Maclean

Department of Social Medicine
University of Edinburgh

Routledge & Kegan Paul
London and Boston

First published in 1974
by Routledge & Kegan Paul Ltd
Broadway House, 68-74 Carter Lane,
London EC4V 5EL and
9 Park Street,
Boston, Mass. 02108, U.S.A.
Printed in Great Britain by
Northumberland Press Limited
Gateshead
© Una Maclean 1974
ISBN 0 7100 7751 3 (C)
      0 7100 7752 1 (P)
Library of Congress Catalog Card No. 73 - 86576

For Aysha

Contents

Preface

At a time when professional opportunities and willingness for experiment and initiative have never been greater nurses today have a wide range of choices open to them. Within the hospitals there is increasing specialisation but this is balanced by a complementary development of community care, requiring nurses to move between hospital and community, to participate in the work of general practice and to co-operate with the staff of complex new health centres.

It has not been customary hitherto to offer courses in the social sciences to nurses in their initial period of training, but both the nature and the conditions of modern nursing practice now contribute to make some introduction to sociology desirable. Many of the illnesses which nurses help to treat or try to prevent have a social component and the nurse's skills will be incomplete without some comprehension of her patients' social settings. It is important that she should appreciate that becoming ill is a social process, involving other people besides the actual patient who confronts her, and that social rules and roles will influence patients' reactions to symptoms and their responses to care. The changes in the structure of the health service are integrating hospital and community services and patients may be discharged early. But the experience of hospitalisation can still be traumatic for the individual, and families may be unprepared for a sick member. If continuity of care is to mean anything nurses will have to bear the social consequences of illness constantly in mind, since it is often nurses, rather than doctors, who have most contact with the sick person. Nurses ought to understand the full meaning of patienthood.

But there is another sense in which a sociological perspective can help the nurse, and this is in regard to her own position In a scene which is constantly shifting and changing, where she may have to alter her roles or act on many different stages, it is helpful to study the development of the nursing profession and of the health services. Such a study may contribute to her understanding and increase her satisfaction in her chosen field.

There are numerous excellent introductory texts on sociology which can be recommended to nurses. But nurses also need material which is specifically relevant to their own work situation and most of the available literature on medical or nursing sociology to date has come from North America where the organisation of health care is very different from our own.

This book was conceived and written to fill a gap in the sociology of the contemporary British nursing scene. It is intended as an introduction to the sociology of nursing and it centres on the triad of nurse, patient and doctor. The accompanying bibliographies should open up vistas of wider and more comprehensive reading and the questions following each chapter may be an aid to pupils and tutors. As this is meant to be a book for people in practical situations, I have tried to minimise jargon and to concentrate on what may be helpful to nurses in their daily encounters with patients and medical staff.

My thanks are due to Miss C. M. Fraser, Principal Health Visitor Tutor of the Queen Margaret College, and to Miss E. C. Thomas, Community Nurse Teacher at the District Nurse Training Centre. It was whilst talking to them and teaching their students that I first realised the value of sociology for different branches of the profession.

Professor Margaret Scott Wright, of Edinburgh University Department of Nursing Studies and Miss M. G. Auld, Matron of the Simpson Memorial Maternity Pavilion,

Edinburgh Royal Infirmary have also been most helpful, and I have benefited from discussions with Miss Elizabeth West of the Scottish Nursing Staffs Committee. I should, however, make it clear that the opinions expressed in this book are my own.

The text was virtually completed before the publication of the Briggs Committee Report, but I have endeavoured to add some reference to its breadth of scholarship and well-considered recommendations for the future of the nursing profession.

Finally I should like to thank Miss Carol Brown, Miss Louise McAdam and Mrs Eda Broadie for secretarial assistance, Miss Norah Parker for finding innumerable books and reports, and my extended family for their forbearance.

UNA MACLEAN

1 The relevance of sociology to nursing

Relevance of sociology to understanding of contemporary patients and nurse's own social and professional situation; the changing spectrum of disease; comparisons between sociology and anthropology; methods of sociological enquiry; subject matter of sociology; role theory; role playing in personal encounters; ascribed and achieved roles; social stratification and social class; reference groups; the family, its purpose, form and cultural variants; socialisation and the family.

The relevance of sociology

The relevance of sociology to nursing has never been greater than today when the role of the nurse is being widely questioned. What is the special characteristic of nursing as a human activity, how does it differ from the kinds of care provided by other professionals, in what directions will nursing develop, how should nurses be trained, how should nursing be related to the wide variety of hospital and community services for health and welfare? At a time of great changes in our own system of medical care these questions are being urgently raised and upon their answers much will depend, both for nurses themselves and for all their potential patients.

For it should never be forgotten that the existence of patients is the reason for any system of nursing and medical care. Although this may seem self-evident it can be partially lost sight of at times when attention is focussed upon the structure or working of one profession.

1

Changing spectrum of disease

We live in an age when medical advances have altered the entire spectrum of illness, eliminating some diseases entirely and greatly modifying others. In the course of this remarkable progress entire groups of people who might formerly have died are now left alive and this admirable result has actually generated fresh problems for society generally and for doctors and nurses in particular. For example, we have been enormously successful, in the Western world, in reducing infant mortality but, in consequence, more deformed babies survive. At the opposite end of the age range, we have been left with a very large proportion of elderly people in our population and this has happened at a time when, for other reasons, there are not enough middle-aged people to support them. The two extremes of life, the very young and the very old, now make most calls upon the medical services. Looked at in another way, we can contrast the needs of the acutely ill with those of the chronically disabled. Our society has a very heavy burden of disability, which the able-bodied must in some sense bear, through the provision of services. Then, in spite of our medical wizardry, there are still certain major, intractable diseases which we cannot cure, like some cancers and heart disease, nor do we as yet know how to prevent them. On the other hand, many conditions can be avoided, or can be benefited by early treatment, whilst others can be greatly ameliorated by appropriate medical and nursing care.

So the patients of today are different from those of yesterday and the conditions from which they suffer are very closely tied up with the structure of society generally and with their own social environments. This is abundantly so in the case of small infants and the aged, but it also applies to every other group of patients one can mention.

If the nurse is to utilise her skills to the best advantage she must see her patients in their social setting and, if she is to understand her own position in the total system of medical care, she needs some information about how medicine and nursing have developed. In both these broad and important areas of interest sociology can supply valuable insights. Sociology tries to explain peoples' actions and endeavours to make sense of some of the apparent confusions and contradictions of their lives.

The lives of both nurses and patients have many facets apart from their common involvement with illness. The sick and those who care for them are simultaneously involved in all kinds of other human relationships and associations which are usually of paramount significance to the people concerned and which incidentally affect their reactions to the medical encounter. For example, nurses have a social life which means a great deal to them; they may be contemplating marriage, they may want to work near a boy-friend or near their own home; similarly, patients in hospital cannot be fully understood in isolation from their families and the social circumstances which they have left and to which they will return. So some knowledge of social groupings outside medical institutions is essential, so that nurses may be able to view their own situation in proper perspective, and appreciate those aspects of the patient's position which affect his response to ill health.

One special reason for the current relevance of sociology to nursing has to do with the fact that nursing nowadays is by no means confined to a hospital setting but is also increasingly practised within the wider community. District nurses, health visitors, nurses attached to a general practice, midwives following up mothers and babies who have recently been discharged from hospital, nurses in industry, nurses on cruise ships, private nurses and nurses going overseas will be working among groups of people whose behaviour is not nearly so orderly and organised as that of rows of tidy patients in identical hospital beds. Nurses in such varied circumstances in the outside world

3

may have problems in defining for themselves and others what their precise function is and how they fit in to other organisations. They will also encounter all sorts of other helping agents in society, voluntary workers, probation officers and, especially, social workers whose work seems, in some respects, closely similar to their own. The person who regards herself as 'simply a nurse' may discover that a mere matter of names is more complicated than she had ever imagined and that she ought to be aware of how the public regard these associated professions and occupations.

Finally, in whatever setting she works, the nurse will almost certainly find that she forms one corner of an eternal triangle. Just as the nurse cannot operate without a patient, so she is unlikely ever to work without being in some relationship, however remote, to a doctor. Doctors and nurses share a reliance upon the existence of patients as the justification for their own occupations; neither the nature of the relationship between nurse and patient nor the public image of nursing can be properly understood without reference to doctors and the medical profession. So the sociology of nursing involves not only the sociology of the patient (what it means to be a patient) but also the sociology of doctors as a group, because how the doctor views his world makes a profound difference to the position of the nurse in her own private universe.

There are a number of different approaches to the study of human behaviour. Two subjects which are closely related to sociology are psychology and anthropology. But, while psychology is mainly concerned with individual responses, social anthropology has more in common with sociology and so it is appropriate to consider its material and methods briefly.

Sociology and anthropology

Sociology tends to concentrate upon aspects of life in 'developed' societies, countries which have many industries, a high level of education for everyone and a relatively high standard of living. Our own country, others in Western Europe and most of North America are examples of such societies. Anthropology, on the other hand, has hitherto been mainly involved with the study of 'underdeveloped' or 'developing' societies, that is to say, parts of the world which are economically much less advanced and in which people's way of life has remained fairly stable. This can only be a broad generalisation, since most traditional societies are in the process of being modified and anthropologists frequently study the effect of changes upon societies which are encountering aspects of twentieth-century 'progress'. Nevertheless, it is true that anthropologists have hitherto tended to concentrate upon what used to be called primitive peoples, leaving to sociologists the study of communities close at hand.

There are historical reasons for this geographical division of labour, related to Britain's experience as an imperial power during the nineteenth century. When British rule extended over India and much of Africa, colonial officers and missionaries frequently collected detailed accounts of the customs pertaining in the parts of the world in which they were stationed. Such descriptions, which tend now to sound very prejudiced and sensational, constituted some of the first essays in anthropology. Colonial district officers held positions of authority in their administrative areas; they were admitted to all the important local occasions, public ceremonies, feasts and funerals, celebrations and sacrifices, as well as being privileged to observe at close quarters many of the domestic details of ordinary people's lives. In the hot countries of Asia and Africa, much of life is lived out of doors in the full public view and, even for a foreigner, it is fairly easy to observe what is going on.

Methods of enquiry

This leads to another difference between sociologists and anthropologists, namely their chosen methods of study. Anthropologists usually depend upon what is termed 'participant observation', meaning that they go and stay for some time among the people whom they wish to understand, learning their language, living in similar circumstances, eating the same food and so on. They try as far as possible to merge into the local background and to become accepted by the tribe or group whom they are investigating, hoping thereby to disturb peoples' normal way of behaving as little as possible. It is of course difficult for someone with a white skin to go unnoticed in a culture where everyone else is coloured. But, in a sense, anthropologists can benefit from the very fact of their obvious difference, because they can thereby convey the fact that they are not personally involved in any of the conflicts and disputes which are going on locally. Although they may be sharing many of the material aspects of life, they remain essentially outsiders, who do not constitute any threat to the established social order.

However, over many parts of the world, anthropology is now tending to give way to sociology. Even in the developing countries of Africa, students of human social behaviour prefer to be regarded as sociologists or economists rather than be identified with anthropology, which retains overtones of colonialism and a patronising attitude to what were once openly regarded as 'savage cultures'. As has been said already, few societies in Africa or Asia or South America remain as 'simple' and unspoilt as formerly. Machine technology, an economy based on money, consumer goods in the form of transistor radios, cars, bicycles, and sewing machines, to say nothing of the impact of modern medicine, are all rapidly transforming traditional societies throughout the world. Then there are problems to do with the disappearance of first hand sources of information about traditional cultures. Anthropologists used to rely upon old men's memories for tales of how people lived in the days of their youth but, as the old men die, much of this unwritten lore is lost for ever, since young people have been brought up, literally, in a very different school. So new methods have to be used to study the changing societies of the developing world, just as new methods are needed in our own countries.

Indeed when anthropologists or sociologists wish to investigate their own societies, they may encounter special obstacles. Although they will not need to learn a new language and although they ought to be superficially familiar with the people they are studying, no one will automatically grant them privileged access. To other people they may simply appear as inquisitive neighbours whose desire to pry into private affairs may be viewed with suspicious hostility.

Moreover, in cold or temperate climates people live inside their homes, not in the full public view, as in the tropics and, once they retreat inside, their doors are closed to strangers. The student of society cannot sidle up and contemplate family life in action as he might in a native compound where the cooking and washing, the feeding of infants and the scolding of toddlers is all proceeding noisily in the backyard. Our own domesticity is enclosed, an Englishman's home is his castle, as the saying goes, and permission to enter and observe will have to be specifically requested and formally granted.

Without prior preparation, the sociologist's work cannot be scientific and precise, and many sociological enquiries are carried out by means of special surveys, using sets of questions which have been carefully planned and rehearsed beforehand. Prior permission to visit a home is often ensured by letter, and then interviews are carried out at times which are convenient to the individual or family concerned.

Some sociologists working in Western societies do

7

employ the anthropological method of participant observation and temporarily identify with the society which interests them. The American sociologist Erving Goffman, who has frequently used this technique, once spent a year in a large mental hospital with his real purpose kept a secret from all but the top management. During this time, whilst he was ostensibly a minor member of the staff, he had an unparalleled opportunity to contemplate the institutional world from the patients' angle and to understand the devices by which they made their restricted circumstances meaningful and tolerable.

In this country, sociologists interested in factory conditions or in the life of small communities have often participated in the social activities which they were observing. The success of this method largely depends upon maintaining anonymity, since otherwise people may be inclined to modify their customary behaviour. They may tend to conform to what they imagine the resident sociologist expects of them, concealing reactions which they would prefer a stranger not to see. In practice, sociologists often combine questionnaire surveys with direct observation, as it is inadequate and impractical to rely upon only one method of collecting information.

Subject matter of sociology

The sociological viewpoint can be taken on many different subjects. Thus, political sociology has to do with people's voting behaviour and their reactions to the processes of government, while the sociology of education takes into account the influence of various social factors upon educational opportunities and achievements. In addition, social psychology, social psychiatry and social medicine are all related to medical sociology. These terms all imply the use of sociological methods and insights in different areas of human behaviour, and the divisions between them are a convenient way of dealing with what is a very wide territory. Such divisions may suggest that events and things in the real world are already separated in themselves, whereas the divisions are actually in the minds of the people who make them.

It is easier to regard sociology generally as being the study of people's behaviour in groups, groups of all kinds, large and small, casual or permanent, groups of which people are very conscious as well as those of which they may scarcely be aware. Thus, much of sociology is concerned with the human family, a group whose form and composition varies from one part of the world to another and from one set of people to another but which does have common features and functions wherever it is studied. The family will be referred to repeatedly in this book, since not only does it affect all our lives but it profoundly influences the way in which people react in relation to illness.

But we all belong to innumerable other human groupings besides the family, such as schools, clubs, professional training courses and college classes; we are parties to friendships; we are members of theatre audiences and holiday crowds; we have been brought up in a village; we may live in a hostel; we briefly join fellow travellers in a bus or a train; we engage in countless casual encounters in shops and streets. In addition there are wider groupings, some of which we may take for granted but which nevertheless influence our behaviour and the possible range of our choices and actions. Examples of such larger groups are race, nationality, our own occupation and that of our parents, our age and our sex.

Society consists of people who are in some kind of relationship with one another, they may be co-operating or they may be acting for their own ends. But, if they are members of any social unit, for whatever purpose, they will all be playing particular parts as they inter-act with one another. These similes from the world of the theatre, like 'playing parts' and 'acting', can be very useful when we start to study the behaviour of groups of people.

9

Role theory

'Role' is another word or concept from the theatre which sociologists frequently employ, because it helps to sum up and describe an important feature of social relationships. The parties to any mutual relationship, such as father and son, husband and wife, nurse and patient, or the members of larger groups such as the guests at a wedding or the students at a graduation ceremony, for example, all expect the others to behave in a particular manner. There are accepted ways of doing things, conventions which everyone knows and unwritten sets of rights and obligations. If a person performs his side of a bargain, if he carries out the tasks expected of him, he expects that the others will respond in turn by fulfilling their proper obligations towards him.

This sounds somewhat deliberate and formal but, in practice, our inter-personal behaviour is not self conscious. We are usually so familiar with the rules of social intercourse that we take them for granted. It may require a foreigner to notice the curious features of a society different from his own; indeed an outsider or stranger of any kind is often placed in conspicuous and embarrassing situations precisely because he is not aware of the local conventions and cannot automatically behave in the manner which is expected of him.

Many examples of role playing can, for example, be observed in the behaviour of people at a busy railway station. Some of those present will be in family groups, or friends seeing others off, or people being effusively greeted as they have just come off a train; the attention of the members of all these small social groups is largely concentrated upon one another and upon their immediate aims. As they play out their familiar small dramas of welcome or parting their behaviour is unlikely to attract undue remark from passers by. The same applies to station employees, each with clear roles to play and functions to fulfil; porters, ticket collectors and the like, everyone knows what is expected of him and treats each one accordingly. Paradoxically, it can be the person on their own, who is not for the moment a member of any group, who may have to be most circumspect about the impression which they are creating upon others.

Consider for instance a girl who has arranged to meet her friend in the station. She will arrive briskly, taking up her stance beneath the station clock with an air of attentive expectancy. From time to time she will glance up at the clock or consult her own wrist watch, or she may take a few steps forward, peering anxiously into the crowd. Eventually her expression will convey impatience, alternating with resignation. All these changes of expression, the little sallies into the crowd, the time checks and so on, are signals sent out for the benefit of anyone who may be watching, and all meaning, 'I am someone waiting for a friend'. She is acting it out, playing the role of a person waiting for a friend, just as though she were performing in a charade.

It is important that she should go through these motions and make her intentions clear because, in our society, it is not considered proper for people simply to do nothing, to hang about, to loiter. Indeed a woman has to be extra careful lest her solitary presence in a public place is misconstrued. Her sex role as well as her 'waiting for a friend' role come into the picture and she must clearly convey, by her demeanour and small gestures, that she is all dressed up with somewhere to go, even if she is going nowhere at that precise moment. By conveying a sense of her relationship to someone absent she contradicts any improper suggestion of availability to those present.

But even men cannot be caught lounging too casually in a busy place, or at a late hour, with no obvious purpose or they may be investigated by the police for possibly 'loitering with intent', as if their intention was certain to be evil. They must convey an impression of purposeful

11

activity even if they are actually doing nothing, and the person who disregards these social expectations may be taken for a vagabond, a potential thief, a drug peddler, or so mentally disturbed as to know no better.

The judgment of other people on a solitary individual or on a newcomer to an existing group is built up from a multitude of small clues emanating from their behaviour and appearance. When we encounter someone for the first time, if the meeting has not been preceded by a detailed introduction, we have to depend largely upon superficial visual information in our first effort to effect a quick categorisation and to fit the newcomer into some existing pigeon-hole. Until we have summed up what kind of person they are and decided what their role must be we will not know how we should behave towards them. Uniforms are obviously very useful aids to the recognition of roles, but this is only the case for those who are aware of their significance; moreover, only a minority of us wear a definite uniform. But a person's general manner of dressing, their hair style, the clothes they choose or are obliged to wear, are all indicators to others of their social standing and purpose. Once a particular mode of dress and length of hair has become associated in the public or official mind with undesirable or anti-social behaviour, innocent young people who affect these fashions may find to their indignation that they are under suspicion or even arrest.

Ascribed and achieved roles

Social roles can be conveniently divided into two types, those which are ascribed and those which are achieved. By ascribed roles are meant those which are allocated to people at birth; we cannot choose our sex, or our kin or our age. But roles which are achieved come about as the result of personal effort and depend upon a conscious decision on the part of the individual concerned to undertake some kind of training, to attempt a specific performance or aspire to a special position. The roles of nurse and doctor, for example, are achieved, they have been reached through a process of training and by passing through prescribed tests and rituals.

Societies differ in the importance they attribute to ascribed roles as compared to achieved roles. In certain parts of the world, the fact that one is a woman restricts and determines experience in virtually every sphere of life. It may be a cause of initial disappointment to parents who have desired a son; it can mean that from the age of six onwards, the small girl is entirely occupied with female domestic tasks, starting by minding younger brothers and sisters and proceeding, through eventual marriage, to the constant bearing and rearing of her own children. The sex role will effectively deny her participation in the entire range of activities which are open to young boys and adult men and will clearly dictate and delimit all her social activities. In parts of many modern societies, by contrast, the roles of men and women are becoming increasingly less differentiated. In Britain today fathers will often mind the children and do the shopping, they will prepare meals on occasions, some will even sew on buttons and wash shirts. In our society women are admitted to occupations (achieved roles) which were once exclusively male preserves. But a complete and permanent reversal of accepted sex roles is still regarded with suspicion. A man who opts for permanent unemployment and housework whilst his wife acts as the breadwinner is viewed with strong disfavour by most people. It does not seem 'right' that this should occur. So, even in Britain, sex is still a basic role and the one which determines the achievement of many other roles by women, effectively forbidding them senior positions in certain occupations and professions, excluding them from certain clubs, reducing their average earnings, and so on.

In contrast to basic roles are others described as general ones, which are associated with special privileges and obligations. They confer distinct advantages, but they also carry with them expectations of a particular standard of behaviour. This is clearly seen in relation to the roles of doctor and nurse, for example, where the public expects a moral code to operate and where self-interest is always supposed to take second place to service. It is the constant anticipation of altruism that gives special significance to the rare threat of a strike by nurses or doctors. Similarly, immoral behaviour on the part of individual doctors or nurses, transgressing the strict code of professional ethics, is liable to receive severe punishment. These healing roles are immensely important, both to individual patients and to society as a whole, and so the occupants of the roles are expected to conform to strict rules. Doctors and nurses are allowed privileged access to the bodies and minds and private lives of individuals and they must respect the unique social positions which they hold. If they do fall short of professional expectations, retribution may take the form of expelling an offender altogether from occupancy of the role, thereby depriving him of its privileges and respect.

General roles such as these are highly regarded by society, because their performance vitally affects the well-being of so many other people, and those who do achieve such respected positions discover that they are encompassed by their professional obligations to a degree which is unknown to the occupants of humbler roles. By contrast, a hairdresser or a factory worker occupies a role which is largely independent of the rest of their daily life and does not interfere with or impinge upon the performance of other roles during leisure. The obligations of the job are limited to certain times and places. Moreover, the role may only be temporary, one job being easily left for another and one person easily taking another's place.

Social stratification

In our society, occupational roles can be ranged on a
scale according to the prestige which is accorded to them.
This forms the basis of our system of social stratification
or division of people according to social class. All societies
have ways of classifying their members and dividing one
category of people from another. In some communities,
such as India, for example, the important factor may be
descent: people are born into a particular caste which sets
severe limits on their whole mode of life, their social relations and their possible occupations. In parts of the world,
race effectively segregates people in the same manner as
caste, rendering certain positions and privileges inaccessible to the members of the race which is deemed locally
to be inferior. Negroes in America and coloured people in
South Africa suffer social disadvantages which may be
crippling to the individuals concerned.

The system of social class divisions in Britain is based
largely upon occupation and the classification of occupations has become increasingly elaborate. Before the
Industrial Revolution there was much less division of
labour than there is today and, in some country areas, it
was possible for large families or for small communities
to be virtually self supporting, themselves producing the
food, clothing, shelter and simple commodities which they
required for their own use. But a highly developed modern
economy depends upon the multiplication of numerous
separate processes of production, with the development of
a vast number of separate skills and jobs, each with their
own clear specifications and rewards. In the general public
esteem some occupations are rated more highly than others
and the way in which they are ranged or ranked has proved
to be a convenient and useful way of classifying them.
Occupation is easy to ascertain, it largely determines a
person's style of life and, within limits, his income. The
Registrar General's classification, which is frequently em-

The relevance of sociology to nursing

ployed in sociological and medical studies, distinguishes five social classes ranging from people holding professional and managerial posts, in Social Class I, to those in unskilled manual occupations in Social Class V.

Social status or standing is, however, often decided in specific instances by other attributes as well as occupation. A person's family connections, their accent, their own educational level and the school to which they send their children, their type of housing, the make of car they own, and the variety of holidays they favour, may all enter into other people's assessment of their precise position on the social scale. Although these attributes are frequently associated, a high income does not necessarily confer high social status and people earning the same amount of money may legitimately be regarded as belonging to different social classes. A worker on a North Sea oil rig, for example, though financially very well rewarded for a time, would never rank higher than a teacher, nor would a pop star outrank a prime minister in the general esteem.

Ordinary people's ideas of social class may not, however, correspond to the precise subdivisions which sociologists employ. Thus most people tend to regard themselves as either 'middle class' or 'working class' and in some cases this is not related to the question of whether or not their occupation is a manual one. Everyone utilises some kind of personal scale by means of which they grade their associates and neighbours, a scale based upon the values which are deemed important within their own social sphere. Groups with special interests employ whole hierarchies of degrees of importance and social influence which are meaningless to outsiders. Amongst pop fans, one particular group may take passing precedence over all others. The distinctions which obtain among professional criminals imply the existence of underground reference groups of which respectable society knows nothing.

16

Reference groups

This phrase 'reference group' is an important and useful one for sociology as it helps to sum up the idea of the differences which exist between various people's standards of behaviour. We frequently measure ourselves and our own achievements against those of others whom we admire and whom we would like to resemble. They form our reference group, they are the groups with which we wish to be identified as closely as possible. A budding athlete may have certain well known amateurs as his reference group and he may model not only his sporting life but also his private existence upon what he knows of his heroes. Other adolescents may earnestly wish to emulate the swash-buckling activities of Hell's Angels, or may adopt, by contrast, the mild, mystical demeanour and casual garb of obscure religious sects. If the behaviour of any of these distinct groups of young people is judged solely upon the basis of the conventional standards of the majority, much of the significance of their activities will be missed, because it does not take into consideration one of the primary influences upon their lives.

The family

So far, a number of recurring sociological concepts have been briefly touched upon, to do with the roles people play in society, the rules by which their actions are regulated and the various social groups of which they form a part. Since the family has such a profound influence on behaviour, it deserves extra attention in this necessarily short introduction.

The human family, in one form or another, has existed since the dawn of history and, in spite of the gloomy prognostications of some latter-day prophets, there is little sign of its imminent demise. For the majority it constitutes the most important primary group in society, consisting of

17

a group of people in a face-to-face relationship linked together by reason of their common interests and their common abode. In these respects it has the characteristics of what sociologists mean by a community. However, by virtue of the fact that a family is formed for certain specific purposes, it also constitutes an organisation, held together to achieve purposes which are important to society as a whole. So, as well as being a community which totally encloses its younger members, the family is also an association of individuals for particular ends. The central purpose of the family is the propagation and rearing of children and, to this end, every society institutes some kind of regulation of sexual behaviour to afford a degree of stability and continuity and to provide a satisfactory environment.

The form of the family has changed enormously in the course of history, from the time when tribal loyalties were paramount and the family could satisfy all human needs, to the present time when, in our own part of the world, it is now a unit of limited size and with diminished functions. However, anthropologists describe family structures which, even at the present time, differ widely from our own. There are many societies, for example, which are polygamous. In these, the family organisation permits more than one wife per husband or, more rarely, more than one husband per wife. Differences also exist in relation to the initial mating arrangements and in the degree to which individuals are allowed to choose their own partners or must submit to this choice being made by their elders. Then there are local variations in regard to the people who live together within the family home, whether they are simply husband and wife and their children, as in the 'nuclear' family with which we are familiar, or whether several married brothers or sisters with their children form parts of one 'extended' family.

Not only has the family varied over time and across cultural barriers but it also changes constantly in the course

18

of any one person's experience. Thus most of us begin life as children in our family of origin, as it is called; growing up, we ourselves eventually proceed to form a new family, through some form of accepted public ritual, a marriage. This new family then progresses through a number of separate stages.

To begin with, before any children are born, there is the nuptual stage, when the couple are getting to know one another and are trying to define and establish their new position in society. With the arrival of children, the child rearing stage begins and this has the effect of converting the family into a much more definite social unit and establishing it in the larger community in an unmistakable manner. At this point, the roles of the marriage partners change from being simply those of husband and wife to being also those of mother and father; their responsibilities increase and the expectations of others regarding their behaviour alter and expand. The stage during which the children are being born and brought to maturity is not only an extremely busy and demanding time for the parents, it is the time during which the primary functions of the family are being fulfilled. Because, in spite of changes and variations, the family remains essentially a group in which the sex relationship is regulated for the purposes of providing a stable background for the bearing and rearing of children.

Whenever the family is studied it is characterised by these three features: first, a mating relationship which is recognised and approved by the rest of society; second, some kind of shared economic provision for children; third, a common dwelling or home. Society is inevitably involved in the way in which individual families bring up their offspring since the very existence and future of any society depends, in the first place, upon the survival of its children and, second, upon the extent to which children adopt or adapt to the culture of their own society.

Socialisation

The process whereby children are taught what are the proper ways of behaving, both within the small family and in the wider society is called socialisation. It involves learning all manner of things, behaviour at mealtimes, the correct disposal of excreta, the complexities of language, the respect they must pay to different adults and the ritual responses they must make to gifts and greetings. In the course of socialisation children slowly learn how to be socially acceptable, and how to restrain their natural reactions in favour of behaviour which their parents and other adults approve. Very importantly, socialisation also involves reactions to pain and illness.

Manners and modes of acting which are learnt very early in life become habits which are extremely tenacious and persistent, so that it is possible to discover traces of distant childhood lessons and experiences in the behaviour of elderly people and patients. The sociological significance of the family, therefore, extends right throughout life, affecting sick and well alike. At times of illness the effects of the family become especially significant, influencing a person's initial responses to his condition, determining his dependence upon continuing nursing care and the prospects of his ultimate recovery. Those who are closely supported by kin are much better off than people who, for one reason or another, are solitary. The position of the lonely old person in our society is potentially dangerous, as they are more than usually liable to illnesses and disabilities, some of which can be greatly eased by adequate medical surveillance. Another group lacking adequate support in our society are unmarried mothers. The many social difficulties which they encounter, compounded of economic hardship, housing difficulties and social ostracism, rebound to the disadvantage of their children. Illegitimate children have a much higher risk of dying in the first year of life than do those who are part of a normal family. Other instances of the effect of the family on health will be given later in this book, as the theme of the social setting of sickness is further developed.

Although it has been necessary, in a short introductory chapter, to simplify a great deal and to select topics from the wide field of sociology, there are many books available which explore the subject at much greater depth. It would be quite wrong to suggest, for example, that families in Britain all behave alike. A little exploration of the literature will demonstrate the wide divergences which can be found in the ways of life of people living relatively close together and the regional differences which exist in many aspects of social behaviour.

Questions

1 Describe what a sociological enquiry might entail, in terms of prior preparations, personal involvement and the numbers of people investigated.
2 How can a knowledge of sociology contribute to your understanding of your present occupation?
3 How would you summarise the universal characteristics of the family?
4 List some aspects of socialisation in children which might affect later reactions to illness.
5 What do you understand by the term 'social class'?
6 What is the official basis for social class, as used by sociologists in Britain?

Further reading

BANTON, MICHAEL (1965) *Roles: An Introduction to the Study of Social Relations*, Tavistock Publications, London.
BERGER, PETER L. (1963) *Invitation to Sociology: A Humanistic Perspective*, Penguin Books, Harmondsworth.
BUTTERWORTH, ERIC and WEIR, DAVID (1970) *The Sociology of Modern Britain: An Introductory Reader*, Fontana Books, Collins, London.

The relevance of sociology to nursing

GOFFMAN, ERVING (1959) *The Presentation of Self in Everyday Life*, Anchor Books, Doubleday, New York.

INKELES, ALEX (1965) *What is Sociology? An Introduction to the Discipline and Profession*, Prentice Hall, New York.

SPROTT, W. J. M. (1963) *Human Groups*, Penguin Books, Harmondsworth.

TURNER, CHRISTOPHER (1969) *Family and Kinship in Modern Britain*, Routledge & Kegan Paul, London.

WILLMOTT, P. and YOUNG, M. (1960) *Family and Class in a London Suburb*, Routledge & Kegan Paul, London.

YOUNG, M. and WILLMOTT, P. (1962) *Family and Kinship in East London*, Penguin Books, Harmondsworth.

II Becoming a patient

Historical perspectives; the sick role in contemporary society; cross-cultural comparisons of beliefs regarding sickness; continued persistence of old attitudes; contrasting behaviour in sickness according to sub-cultural groups, especially social class; further factors influencing sickness behaviour, age, sex, educational level, experience, availability of treatment; the universality of symptoms; contingent factors determining decision to seek professional help.

Historical perspectives on illness

At all times and in all cultures illness has been part of human experience and people have been obliged to come to terms with it. Consequently we find accounts of an enormous variety of different ways of dealing with illness, both from past civilisations and periods of history and also from contemporary societies in other parts of the world which have their own characteristic ways of responding to disease, disability and death.

It is worth contemplating some of these historical and cultural variations on the theme of illness, because it is all too easy to take it for granted that our own way of combating disease is, if not unique, at least so patently superior that it is likely to be accepted everywhere. The skills and methods of modern medicine and its practitioners can undoubtedly claim credit for many remarkable successes. But there exist broad areas of human belief and behaviour which influence personal health for better or worse and which are independent of different methods of treatment and, unless nurses are aware of these deeply entrenched attitudes and habits, they may never come to understand their patients completely. Further, without a knowledge of their patients' outlook, nurses may not utilise the best means of educating the public about health or the management of sickness. Whilst this is of importance to nurses in practice anywhere, it is more than ever relevant for those who have occasion to work among unfamiliar people and places.

It seems as if every society of which we have knowledge has recognised the special position of the sick and has made some kind of provision for its diseased or injured members. Evidence from places as far apart as Western Germany and Peru shows that, even in pre-historic times, there were specialists able to undertake hazardous operations on bones, such as trephining, cutting a hole in the skull. What we do not know and shall never know, however, is why these operations were done or what were the ideas about the nature of disease held by our earliest ancestors.

The word 'patient' is derived from the Latin for suffering. It denotes a passive condition, a state of relative inactivity, when things happen to a person instead of his being responsible for his own actions. Becoming a patient is not, however, simply a matter of receiving a specific diagnosis from a doctor. It also establishes the patient's occupancy of a well recognised social role. Once someone is regarded by themselves or others as a patient, they are expected to act in a particular manner, they become the recipients of important rights but they also have certain duties. Other people, for their part, must act towards the patient in the appropriate manner and must fulfil certain obligations towards them. Once the 'sick' role has been conferred upon an individual he is thereby enabled, quite legitimately, to give up his customary mode of life for the duration of the illness. In this way society ensures the best possible conditions for his recovery and his return to full functioning as a member of the wider community.

The sick role in contemporary society

The American sociologist Talcott Parsons has summed up the four conditions which characterise the adoption of the sick role in a society like our own. In the first place, the illness must be outside the patient's control, in no sense his own fault. Second, the sick role will allow him exemption from his other roles, with their associated obligations and duties. For example, a man can legitimately give up work and leave his usual family responsibilities to his wife. But, third, the sick role requires that the patient should positively desire to get well, he should not relish the relinquishment of responsibility and, fourth, he has the obligation to seek competent medical help.

We are accustomed to considering the sick as unfortunate people, entitled to sympathetic care and attention, partly because we regard illness as a misfortune which has overtaken someone through no fault of their own. This is, in fact, one of the important pre-conditions which we lay down before permitting a person to adopt the sick role and to receive the special privileges and advantages which go along with patienthood. But the modern view of illness as something fortuitous and blameless is somewhat exceptional and other societies have taken a different attitude to the question.

Previous attitudes to the sick

Looking at the matter historically, it is clear from a study of the Old Testament, for example, that the Israelites judged many diseases to be a punishment, a clear sign of the disapproval of the Almighty and an awful warning of what might befall others similarly tempted to transgress. They even believed that disease could descend upon innocent children, as a result of the misdeeds of their parents or grandparents. For the Jews, serious sickness always represented some kind of mark or stigma, setting

25

the sick person apart from the rest of society, labelled as undesirable, despised and rejected. They were also pre-occupied with detailed procedures for ritual purification, measures intended to remove contagion from contacts who had encountered the sick or wrongdoer.

The ancient Greeks, who were not so preoccupied with ideas of transgression and purity, set great store upon physical and spiritual perfection. In consequence, cripples and those who were obviously deformed occupied an im-paired and inferior status; they were people who had clearly failed in the contest for health, strength and beauty and they could never expect a respected position in the community. Although physicians were highly esteemed, the sick whom they had failed to cure were inevitably classed as second-rate citizens.

It was Christianity which eventually introduced the view of the sick from which most of our current attitudes are derived. Far from regarding sickness as a sign of sin, it saw sin itself as a sickness, demanding a radical cure, whilst the sick themselves occupied a condition of grace and merit. The suffering which disease might entail was regarded as positively valuable, since it could assist some-one to improve his spiritual state and to achieve salvation. Fortunately, it was simultaneously urged that the relief of suffering was a praiseworthy duty. So, the social situation of the sick person was enormously improved, stigma and rejection being replaced by an attitude of benignity and acceptance. Meanwhile the sick were seen to deserve the best of care and attention from physicians, family and neighbours.

The history of medicine recounts the many changes which have taken place, over centuries, in our ideas about the causes of different illnesses, and records many fashions in diagnosis and treatment which seem horrifying today. But all the fearful regimes and mixtures which were pre-scribed for patients in the past seem to have been willingly and gratefully received, as evidence of due care and concern on the part of learned physicians who were as skilled as their times permitted. Patients everywhere are people in need, serious illness always constitutes a crisis, and some kind of treatment is always better than none.

Cultural considerations

There are very large areas of the world which, even today, are so short of doctors, drugs and hospital beds that the impact of modern Western medicine is negligible and people are still obliged to rely upon local beliefs and methods of treatment. These have gradually been built up by traditional medical experts and are widely accepted as representing the best form of help which the patient and his relatives can obtain.

Anthropologists and doctors have collected descriptions from all over the world of complex theories regarding the causes of illness and the actions which patients should take to deal with their misfortune. Many of these ideas seem very strange and even repulsive. But just as our own concepts of medical care are rooted in our own history, related to our system of beliefs, to our religion and our rules regarding inter-personal behaviour, so the apparently curious customs of other cultures are rational and sensible to the people of these different societies.

In many parts of South America, the possible effects of the 'evil eye' are greatly dreaded and mothers may attribute their babies' illnesses to the malevolent glances of strangers. They are convinced that if a very powerful personality casts his gaze upon an individual who is weak or helpless, then symptoms will result. A small, pretty child is thought to be especially vulnerable and in need of protection. Guatemalan Indians consider that, before sickness occurs, an external agent must act upon someone whose body is already in a susceptible condition. This same belief underlies their diagnosis of 'susto' when, they think, someone's soul has been captured by an evil spirit, a situation which

27

can, however, only take place if the victim has just suffered a severe shock. For example, a person might fall ill after seeing a snake. So although the diagnoses which South American Indians make seem bizarre, the idea behind them is relatively sophisticated. After all, in our bacteriological germ theory of disease we are accustomed to the idea that someone whose 'resistance' has been lowered is more likely to contract an infection.

Throughout tropical Africa the belief that illness can be spiritually caused is practically universal. It is not sufficient for a patient to be told that his disease or accident has come about as the result of pure chance since he will demand to know 'who' was responsible and 'why' it should have occurred at just that time and in precisely that place. The African patient will try to discover some person who is ill-disposed towards him, some ancestor who has been offended, some god whom he has neglected adequately to serve. He requires a particular reason for his particular misfortune. Furthermore, he considers that evil thoughts and wishes can operate upon him from a distance and that certain 'medicines' can be effective even if they never come in contact with his body. He may concoct complicated mixtures which are equivalent to magical charms or potions, and these may be simply poured out upon the ground, or buried, or placed in a chosen spot. But in order to be potent, such mixtures require to be prepared and used to the accompaniment of appropriate 'incantations' or spells. Moreover, there are all kinds of healing specialists in practice, ranging from herbalists to priestly healers equivalent to our psychiatrists, to whom patients may turn for simple advice or for very elaborate treatment.

In northern India a multitude of priests, magicians, exorcists and others are available to treat disease in ways which are familiar and trusted by the local people. Much faith is placed in charms and amulets which parents pathetically hope will protect their small children from the diseases to which so many fall victim. Magical treatments are freely bought and sold in the markets, and people will try a whole succession of remedies and practitioners in their anxious search for cures.

To any of these diverse peoples, in the Americas, in Africa and in India, the common opening remark of our own type of doctor, 'Now tell me what is the matter with you?', sounds absurd. They are all convinced that it is a proper doctor's business to 'know' intuitively what is wrong with his patient and, if he has to do any systematic diagnosing, it is likely to be by a process more akin to astrology or divination than by seeking for physical signs and symptoms.

It is very important, however, not to lose sight of those features which all patients share, whether they are people in Britain, consulting their own familiar general practitioner, or peasants in India attending a noted magician. In the first place, they have confidence in their own local system and their local practitioner. The medical system as they know it is socially sanctioned and it is the acceptable, normal procedure for the people concerned to employ whatever services are available. There are clear expectations as to how the patient and the healing agent should behave towards one another, a concensus in regard to their reciprocal obligations. Moreover, for the patient to embark upon what is deemed the correct procedure for alleviating an illness will often in itself reduce his worry and uncertainty. Once an illness has been named or explained it loses some of its strangeness and terror, whilst the experience of handing it over to an accredited expert is a further great source of reassurance.

Until modern medicine arrives on the scene, traditional methods of dealing with disease may go unchallenged but, in many developing countries nowadays, both systems exist side by side. There is usually a great shortage of personnel, but, although their numbers are small, there are some trained nurses and doctors, and some hospitals and clinics for them to work in. It is not uncommon for workers in the health field to feel a missionary enthusiasm for replacing all the prevailing superstitions with the blessings of scientific medicine and to feel that the matter is merely one of replacing ignorance with knowledge. Faced by evidence of dirt and disease, nurses and doctors have been repeatedly surprised and disillusioned by the reluctance of the local population to adopt new ideas which seem so clearly superior to their own. People are incorrigibly reluctant to modify their own ways of rearing children, unwilling to change their diet or begin boiling their drinking water, persistent in their reliance on weird concoctions, unreliable in their observance of new therapeutic measures. A little time spent studying local medical customs and the beliefs which underlie them will be amply repaid, as the health practitioner will get much better results by gently modifying and adapting old methods than by ruthlessly rejecting them. For example, in a part of rural Ghana when young, trained midwives were first introduced the local women scarcely used their services, preferring instead to patronise the familiar old grandmothers who had traditionally presided over deliveries and who observed all the appropriate rituals and customs. It turned out eventually that these venerable midwives were pleased and proud to be offered a modicum of training. Thus equipped, they were better able in every way to assist the progress of modern obstetrics, since their personal identification with the new system soon brought patients along to the antenatal clinics.

To ignore local beliefs can be to invite failure; thus, in the course of a South African campaign against tuberculosis, one old Zulu patriarch was told that his daughter was spreading the infection among the family. The statement was, in his eyes, tantamount to accusing the girl of being a witch and he promptly withheld permission for the treatment or immunisation of any members of his household.

Persistence of old attitudes

The various historical and cultural concepts of illness which have been mentioned so far could be dismissed as mere curiosities, only of interest to those who have occasion to nurse in remote hospitals or districts overseas However, it is possible to discern traces of old attitudes quite close at hand in our own society, affecting the patients whom we encounter daily.

For example, there is no doubt that certain diseases still carry some degree of stigma and are obscurely felt to represent a punishment for wrongdoing. Veneral disease undoubtedly falls into this category. In addition, disfiguring skin conditions arouse the feeling that the sufferer, and not merely his skin, must be 'dirty'. Illegitimate children and children of racially mixed parentage often receive scant sympathy from the community, to such an extent that they are more likely to be subject to certain childhood illnesses. There is still a vague feeling that the children are suffering from their parents' sins.

Society's attitude towards the physically disabled clearly contains the implication that such people are spoiled or impaired, and they frequently have to accept second-rate treatment and status. The mentally subnormal, forever incapable of cure, suffer the worst consequences of permanent impairment, their predicament being made worse by the fact that the very nature of their disability prevents them from intelligent protest.

Whilst we may laugh at witchcraft or the evil eye, we ourselves are aware that illnesses can, in an important sense, be brought about by other people. It is neither superstitious nor absurd to recognise the influence of social relationships upon the nature and course of personal sickness. Just as the help and sympathy evoked by an illness can draw the members of a family closer together and can contribute to cure, so neglect, unkindness and cruelty can all exacerbate ill health. To take a simple but important example, elderly people living alone, without the social support of a family, are notoriously liable to serious illness.

Villagers in India or Africa may resort to a variety of protective charms, but, similarly, ordinary people in our own neighbourhood go along to the local chemist for multivitamins or protective tonic mixtures as soon as winter threatens. Meanwhile, the continuing, half-serious belief in magical influences is evidenced by the popularity of astrology. The sale of all kinds of curious devices, such as slimmers' wheels, electrical reducing belts, bust developers and enveloping plastic garments bear witness to people's unfailing faith in wonderful objects trusted to render them miraculously more socially acceptable. Meanwhile the growing popularity of herbalists and 'health food' stores attests to a wide demand for medicaments outside the orthodox pharmacopoeia.

We have mentioned the sociologist's description of the processes which are entailed in becoming a patient and being given the status of a sick person, permitted to rely upon the attention of others. In a society like our own, which sets great store upon hard work and achievement, to be idle is seen as a rare privilege, something which definitely ought to be discouraged lest too many people seek to take advantage of it. The picture of the 'good patient' is certainly familiar to nurses. It means someone who wholeheartedly co-operates with the staff in a sincere effort to get better, takes his medicine, obeys all orders and is consistently humble, grateful and uncomplaining.

Influences on sickness behaviour: sub-culture

However, not all patients fit this description and, even within Western society, different groups of people, or subcultures as they are sometimes called, can have varying views as to how they should behave when ill. Some of the evidence for this has to come from America, where a mixture of immigrant nationalities have contributed to compose the population. A sociologist there, Mark Zborowski, has made a number of interesting observations of the varying reactions to pain of, for example, Italian-American and Jewish-American patients as compared with native-born Americans. When a group of men with spinal diseases in a large New York hospital were observed it was noticed that, on the whole, those of Italian origin reported more symptoms than the others did; they more often declared that the symptoms were making them irritable, and they were more inclined to consider that their symptoms interfered with their social and personal life. But, although they complained very volubly to start with, they were eager to accept whatever medicines were offered and soon became relatively calm and cheerful again. The Jewish-American patients were much less vocal, but they were clearly deeply disturbed about what their illness might mean, in terms of long-term disability. The nurses found them extremely difficult to reassure and had to supervise them carefully, as they were liable not to take their drugs because of ill-founded fears of addiction. Meanwhile, the patients of Anglo-Saxon stock came much closer towards fulfilling the staff's expectations. They evinced only a moderate degree of initial anxiety; thereafter they took an intelligent interest in their diagnosis and treatment and could be relied upon to follow the prescribed regime. In fact they were the 'ideal' patients, whilst the emotional, noisy Italians were liable to be labelled 'psychiatric' cases by nurses who themselves held the prevailing attitudes towards illness of white, Protestant Americans.

An explanation for the differences in these men's reactions in the face of similar circumstances could well lie in the way they had been brought up. Italian families in New York pay great attention to small children, they show them enormous sympathy if they are hurt in any way and allow their feelings unlimited expression. Jewish mothers on the other hand, are renowned for being virtually obsessive about matters of health and hygiene. Not only do they note isolated illness incidents or accidents but they concentrate upon all the means of avoiding ill health and its consequences. Meanwhile, American mothers rear their sons to be 'manly' and 'brave', they do not tolerate undue complaining but they do tend to insist on the child submitting to treatment at once, even if this means no more than the prompt application of sticking plaster. The patients in this particular investigation all lived in a poor, overcrowded area of the Bronx; financially, they were in similar straits, yet they were preserving many elements of the sub-culture from which they were derived and an important part of this culture, transmitted to the children in the course of socialisation, related to behaviour in the event of illness.

Age and sex

Coming closer to home, it has been shown that in Britain there are all kinds of factors which affect the way in which people respond to symptoms and which effectively influence the initial decisions which they make as to whether or not they should seek professional advice. In the first place, there is the influence of age; elderly people, brought up long before the advent of a free health service, may have restricted notions of what constitutes sufficient justification for a consultation. They may be inclined to accept a considerable amount of inconvenience and disability as the inevitable concomitants of ageing, not meriting the attention of a doctor. Their learning and personal experience regarding illness has been very different from that of the young and, just as they often equate existing old people's homes with former workhouses, so they regard the prospect of hospital admission as a terrifying fate.

Sex roles also come into the picture; it is, for example, well known that more women patients than men receive a diagnosis of psychoneurosis. It looks as though, in our society, it may be more acceptable for women than for men to confess to feelings of fear, anxiety and inadequacy and to evince a variety of 'nervous' symptoms.

It might be supposed that a child would learn specifically neurotic ways of reacting from his mother. But those who have looked closely into this matter have found that it is not necessarily the case that an over-protective, worried mother produces the same traits in her children. Although mothers who are conscious of a great deal of stress may be inclined to report more illness in their children, these children, when questioned, are not themselves over-conscious of symptoms or especially intolerant of minor discomforts. Children, it seems, whilst they absorb general attitudes to illness from the wider society in which they are brought up, do not always precisely reflect their mother's responses to actual signs of possible illness. This is in part because the child can depend upon the mother to look after his symptoms in the same way as she looks after other aspects of his life. She takes his troubles upon herself in the same way as the doctor accepts his patients' woes.

Social class

It is a great mistake to imagine that people with symptoms will always seek a doctor's advice, and a further important determinant of their behaviour is social class. Both from Britain and the United States comes evidence to show what a large proportion of common complaints are dealt with by other means than those of professional medicine. For example, a classic American study on the health of 'Regionville' demonstrated the influence of social class upon the decision to go for medical treatment. In this investigation a sample of people were interviewed and asked a number of questions relating to their views on health and illness. Subsequently the answers were sorted according to the social class to which the respondents belonged, whether they were unskilled workers, skilled workers or professional people. When asked whether they considered that certain symptoms required medical attention the answers varied according to social class. Thus, whilst all the professional class were of the opinion that blood in the urine was a symptom sufficiently serious to merit a consultation, only 69 per cent of unskilled workers thought so. Ninety-four per cent of women from the professional class level would seek medical attention if they discovered a lump in their breast, but only 44 per cent of women whose husbands were in unskilled work said that they would consult. Similar class differences emerged in relation to a whole list of other symptoms, such as swelling of the ankles, blood in the stools, loss of weight, shortness of breath and so on, all of these being from a medical point of view potentially serious conditions.

Another section of the same enquiry dealt with the question of proprietary medicines, medicines which could be bought at a chemists or store, and here it was found that people belonging to a lower social class had more of certain 'remedies' in their possession than did the better off. It was interesting that whilst 90 per cent of professional families were in possession of antiseptics, only 51 per cent of the families of unskilled workers kept these at home. When it came to such substances as 'kidney pills' and 'liver pills' and 'stomach medicines', however, the situation was reversed, these being more commonly kept in the homes of the poor.

The relevance of poverty to health behaviour must never be lost sight of when reading accounts of patients' behaviour in America, because the ability to pay for treatment may well be a significant determining factor. When a consultation costs money, people are bound to hesitate and to try various home remedies before putting an additional strain upon limited family budgets. Symptoms for which middle-class people might demand attention may need to be suffered by those in straitened circumstances.

Education

But the social class differences which were observed in this American study were related not simply to income but also to education. Professional people are likely to possess more up-to-date information about medical matters; they read different newspapers; popular magazines will supply them with graphic accounts of the latest medical discoveries; the written word is likely to play a considerable part in forming thier views. By contrast, working-class people will probably depend much more on hearsay and personal experience. So it is not surprising to discover a class contrast in the kinds of proprietary medicines which were kept in different homes and that this contrast actually reflects an historical difference in terms of medical thought. The germ theory of disease, with its concomitant ideas of 'sepsis' and 'antisepsis' is relatively recent. Upper- and middle-class families, imbued with the importance of hygiene, now think in terms of 'destroying germs'. But, before the days of bacteriology, before the importance of antiseptics, people relied upon all kinds of curious concoctions and mixtures which were unscrupulously advertised as being able to cure all ills. The 'Age of Quackery', as it has been called, is now past and both Britain and the United States enforce strict regulations relating to drug advertisements. But, on both sides of the Atlantic, sundry liver pills and stomach mixtures continue to find a ready sale amongst many people whose medical knowledge is limited and outdated. So, whilst income level is important in deciding sickness behaviour, it is not the only relevant social factor.

About the same time that the 'Regionville' study appeared in the States, two general practitioners in Britain published an analysis of the proportion of illness in the population which was being brought to the attention of the medical services. The social situation here was significantly different from that in America because we had established a National Health Service from which everyone was entitled to free medical advice. But it was calculated that only one quarter of all the episodes of illness which occurred in the community ever came to the attention of a general practitioner.

Experience

Evidence from subsequent surveys in this country has shown that, at any time, up to 90 per cent of people possess symptoms of one sort or another. But the mere presence of symptoms does not, in itself, even make people regard themselves as sick, far less dispose them to seek professional advice. Symptoms like cough, breathlessness, headache, indigestion, backache and constipation, and conditions such as colds, are all commonly tolerated and treated at home. Faced with the realisation that it is normal for people to experience some degree of discomfort, some kind of symptomatology, medical sociologists have begun to wonder what it is that does drive people to take the comparatively unusual step of consultation.

One way of visualising this situation is to imagine that disease is like an iceberg, only a small proportion of it is visible above the surface as it were, whilst the greater part remains hidden from the view of doctors and nurses. A great number of the symptoms which people experience daily are trivial, transient and unimportant. They do not constitute signs of serious disease and it is eminently reasonable that they should be patiently borne or mildly medicated. Yet there is no doubt that some illnesses would be much more susceptible to treatment or cure if only people would report them earlier. This is pre-eminently the case, for example, with certain cancers. But it also applies to conditions which, though relatively minor in themselves, can produce increasing handicaps. Old people who fatalistically accept bunions and ingrowing toe nails may ultimately be bedridden and thereby liable to serious illnesses like broncho-pneumonia. Poor mothers in crowded rented rooms may delay seeking advice for their babies' severe colds which may presently develop into fatal chest infections. Stout middle-aged women may cheerfully put up with the breathlessness which obesity entails until their excess weight precipitates heart failure. The topics investigated by medical sociologists are not of merely academic interest, therefore, since they are concerned with the essence of preventive medicine. Health visitors and all nurses who are involved in the community should carry with them a picture of the universality of symptoms and should try to understand what it is that makes some people complain while others suffer in silence.

So far a number of cultural and social factors have been mentioned which are related to the prevailing views of illness held by a particular society, the behavioural norms characteristic of different social classes, the influence of age, sex and personality and the interaction of the potential patient with the existing system of medical care.

Special circumstances

But, in order to acquire a clearer picture of the processes which are at work, it is necessary to look even closer, at the special circumstances surrounding the decision to seek professional advice. Becoming ill is essentially a social affair, other people are involved, both in defining the role and in dealing with its consequences. So it is useful to focus on what takes place in a family when one of its members shows signs of incapacity. This kind of close-up, detailed study has recently been very well done by David Robinson, a medical sociologist in South Wales. Over a period of eighteen months he was in frequent contact with a small number of families containing young children. The mothers kept diaries for him, noting every symptom and what action was taken. There were other aspects to the enquiry, special attitude tests and so on, but the main purpose was to secure the maximum information about the decision making processes involved in dealing with signs of illness.

It turned out that the status of the family member was a very important factor. Thus, tiredness was never regarded as a sign of illness in working-class fathers, being a condition too common for concern. But wives and young children would be suspected of falling sick if they seemed more tired than usual. Going off their food was regarded as an ominous sign in children of any age.

When becoming sick was likely to involve loss of working time and earnings, it was clear that careful calculations were made, based upon detailed social balances of profit and loss. If, for example, the father suffered an injury, his decision as to whether or not to consult the doctor might depend on a number of precise considerations. He would have to reckon upon the possible damage to himself in his employer's eyes which absence from work might occasion. Whereas if he had been in a job for a long time this consideration might scarcely bother him, if he had just taken up a new position he would be anxious to establish a reputation for reliability. Finally, if he was currently out of work he could easily take on 'being ill' as his major social role.

In this connection it is important to note the doctor's role, not simply as a person who makes an individual diagnosis but as someone accepted by society to legitimise, to make legal and proper, the assumption of the status 'sick'. Certification is, in our medical system, the outward and visible sign of having been given the sick role. Moreover, it carries financial rewards. But someone who is unemployed can take to his bed for several days without any doctor's sanction, all he needs is his family's acquiescence in this behaviour. For their part, individual family members usually make their own astute assessments of just how much of the symptomatology of others they can ignore and at what point they will be bound to take

40

someone's complaints seriously. Mothers constanly have to decide whether their toddler's fretfulness derives from tantrums or teething or whether it signals the start of an illness; similarly, on many a morning, they must rapidly make up their minds whether to grant a school child the luxury of a day off, in view of headaches which could bear more relation to the imminence of a test than to the onset of a fever. Husbands have to consider whether their wife's dramatic prostration at the end of a day's washing betokens illness, frustration or frigidity, and wives must, in their turn, calculate whether their husband's inability to mow the lawn needs to be taken as a sign of physical weakness.

An important consideration in respect of any new symptom is how far it is perceived as a threat or danger, how far it is likely to interfere with what a person plans to do or has to do. If it looks as though a condition will seriously disrupt social activities, the person concerned is likely to take prompt action to secure help and relief. This is, of course, notably the case with sudden, acute symptoms; their urgency is betokened by their very nature and they demand immediate attention from all concerned. However, the great bulk of sickness experience is by no means dramatic; on the contrary, it is mildly troublesome or ambiguous, varying in intensity and in the inconvenience which it occasions. In their reactions to feelings of disease or malaise, people will be guided by a great variety of influences. First of all, they will assess the implications of the actual symptoms on the basis of their familiarity. The common cold, as its name implies, causes as a rule the minimum of worry, although it can be an undoubted inconvenience. Symptoms which are common, whose out-come is well known as non-serious, are easily disregarded. But if symptoms persist and if they are intensified their progression may force action. Symptoms which are relatively unfamiliar, such as a bloodstained discharge, may occasion varying reactions, according to a person's memory

41

and experience of similar conditions in other people whom they have known.

The place of formal and informal sources of information has already been mentioned; there exists in our own society as well as in remoter cultures a folk lore of illness. The popular press, largely in the form of advertisements but also in doctors' and nurses' advice columns, turns out a steady stream of snippets of information and misinformation. Meanwhile, any potential patient and their relatives have to weigh up the immediate advantages and disadvantages of 'going sick', what are the risks and possible consequences of delaying advice and treatment as compared with the inconvenience of going to the doctor. In circumstances where the inconvenience may entail real financial hardship there can be a positive disincentive to consultation.

All the time patients and those around them try to make sense of their symptoms, and, in this constant process of definition and redefinition and interpretation, they use quite different criteria from those of the medical professions. Time and again it has been shown that ordinary people's interpretation of common medical terms can be far removed from the meaning which nurses and doctors intend. Patients misunderstand, they fail to hear, they forget, they are anxious, they get confused over details. Most of the community have the minimum of medical knowledge yet, at the same time, they are liable to a multiplicity of symptoms and signs. Becoming a patient is an extremely complicated process and the person who has finally taken or been given the sick role is preoccupied with all kinds of considerations which his medical attendants may find trivial and irrelevant. 'Why should this happen to me?' he wonders. What ever can he have done to deserve such a misfortune, just when he has moved house, or taken on fresh responsibilities? What is going to happen to the children, the car, the business? In any conversation between a new patient and a nurse or doctor there will be a tremendous amount of speculation on the patient's part, ideas of causation—'It must have been a chill. . . .' 'Of course it happened just after a fall. . . .' 'I told him he should never have moved the wardrobe. . . .'

The sociology of the patient is not the sociology of the nurse or doctor; they inhabit different worlds, they use a different language, they are moved by different priorities and interests. Nevertheless, with due care and imagination, all those who encounter patients ought to be able to enter some way into their private worlds and to appreciate the meaning to them of their own condition. Time spent on this exercise will make it more likely that treatments will be accepted and followed and will help relieve the anxieties which most patients endure.

Questions

1 Describe some of the ideas about illness causation which have been held by people remote from us in time or space.
2 List the factors which can influence the reactions of lay people to sudden symptoms. (Remember that their interpretation may be different from your own view, as a nurse.)
3 How can education affect someone's response to the development of an illness?
4 'Doctors and patients speak a different language.' What does this statement mean to you?
5 If you decided to work overseas in a tropical country, what are some of the things you would like to know about the people among whom you intended to work.
6 Give sociological reasons why elderly people may not make adequate use of medical care facilities.
7 How may the circumstances of a child's upbringing modify his reactions to ill health in later life?

Further reading

BENEDICT, RUTH (1966) *Patterns of Culture*, Routledge & Kegan Paul, London.
BLOOM, SAMUEL W. (1963) *The Doctor and his Patient: A*

Sociological Interpretation, Russell Sage Foundation, New York.

BOYLE, CHARLES M. (1970) 'Difference between patients' and doctors' interpretation of some common medical terms', *British Medical Journal*, ii, 286-9.

CARSTAIRS, G. M. (1955) 'Medicine and faith in rural Rajasthan', in *Health, Culture and Community*, ed. Benjamin Paul, Russell Sage Foundation, New York.

FREIDSON, ELIOT (1961) *Patients' Views of Medical Practice*, Russell Sage Foundation, New York.

GORDON, GERALD (1966) *Role Theory and Illness: A Sociological Perspective*, College and University Press, New Haven, Conn.

JACO, E. G. (1958) ed., *Patients, Physicians and Illness*, Free Press, Chicago.

KING, STANLEY G. (1962) *Perceptions of Illness and Medical Practice*, Russell Sage Foundation, New York.

KOOS, E. L. (1954) *The Health of Regionville*, Columbia University Press, New York.

KOOS, E. L. (1959) *The Sociology of the Patient*, McGraw-Hill, New York.

LEY, P. and SPELMAN, M. S. (1967) *Communicating with the Patient*, Staples Press, London.

MACLEAN, UNA (1971) *Magical Medicine: A Nigerian Case-Study*, Allen Lane, The Penguin Press, London.

MECHANIC, DAVID (1964) 'The influence of mothers on their children's health attitudes and behaviour', *Paediatrics, 33*, 444-53.

PARSONS, TALCOTT (1966) 'On becoming a patient', in *A Sociological Framework for Patient Care*, eds J. R. Folta and E. Deck, John Wiley, New York.

PARSONS, T. and FOX, R. (1952) 'Illness, therapy and the modern urban American family', *Journal of Social Issues, 18*.

PAUL, BENJAMIN (1955) ed., *Health, Culture and Community*, Russell Sage Foundation, New York.

PEARCE, EVELYN (1969) *Nurse and Patient: Human Relations in Nursing*, Faber & Faber, London.

READ, MARGARET (1966) *Culture, Health and Disease*, Tavistock Publications, London.

ROBINSON, DAVID (1971) *The Process of Becoming Ill*, Routledge & Kegan Paul, London.

SAUNDERS, LYLE (1954) *Cultural Differences and Medical Care*, Russell Sage Foundation, New York.

SIGERIST, HENRY E. (1960) 'The special position of the sick', from *On the Sociology of Medicine*, ed. M. I. Roemer, M.D. Publications, New York.

SUSSER, M. W. and WATSON, W. (1971) *Sociology in Medicine*, Ch. 2, 'Culture and health', Oxford University Press, London.

ZBOROWSKI, MARK (1966) 'Cultural components in response to pain', in *A Sociological Framework for Patient Care*, eds J. R. Folta and E. Deck, John Wiley, New York.

III The role and image of the nurse

Derivations and family connotations of nursing; early historical references to nurses and midwives; nurse as servant; society's attitudes to dangerous dirt; different prestige levels of bodily service; the nurse in the pre-Nightingale era; the introduction of nurse training in Britain, with the medical and social changes which influenced it; the objectives of nurse training; ways of achieving objectives and changing the outlook of new recruits; the development of the nursing hierarchy; increasing medical specialisation and the division of nursing labour; the establishment of nursing as a profession; the growth of interest in nursing management, its merits and possible pitfalls; recent professional re-orientation towards patient needs; public images of the nurse.

Family connotations of nursing

The word 'nurse' has a simple and noble origin. Ultimately derived from the verb to nourish, it connotes someone who supplies life-giving comfort and support. It is small wonder that nurses are generally thought of as women since, for all of us, our first nurse was our mother, an idealised figure of infinite patience and resource symbolising food and warmth, shelter, security and sympathy, always at hand to meet our every need. The position of the patient is essentially one of dependence and helplessness and the nurse fulfils the complementary function of ministering to the sick, providing for them the elementary supports without which life cannot continue.

Before exploring the complexities of the nurse's role as it has been developed over the course of time, it is necessary to pay tribute to these fundamental aspects of nursing. Because, although nurses have by now specialised and developed their professional capacities in a multiplicity of ways, their practice is still inextricably bound up with the total care of sick patients, and the search for an identity which ignores or minimises their basic reasons for existence is doomed to failure.

Just as the roles of nurse and mother are closely related, so it is the case that most nursing has, until today, taken place within the family. Before hospitals were commonplace the care of the sick usually devolved upon wives and mothers and sisters, aided by such domestic servants as the family could afford. Subsequently, as will presently be shown, the images of both the hospital and the nurse greatly changed, but it was still exceptional for a sick person to require admission to hospital.

The family connotations of the profession are clearly shown in other words associated with nursing; matron, for example is derived from the Latin for mother, whilst sister is a term implying a close relationship from which sex is explicitly excluded. It is no coincidence that the same words, mother and sister, are to be found in women's religious orders because, during the Middle Ages in Europe, the institutional care of the sick was in the hands of the church; a connection which has continued in some Catholic countries to the present day.

Midwife or wet nurse

Nursing has always been closely related to birth and infant care. The local midwife has been a familiar nursing figure in numerous traditional societies; generally an old woman with extensive experience of deliveries, she acted as the repository of female wisdom concerning such matters. In the days before artificial infant foods were invented and when feeding from cup or bottle was highly likely to cause infections, ladies who could afford it might seek to engage a wet-nurse to suckle their baby, if they were unfit or unwilling to rear the child themselves.

For this purpose, a young lactating mother of the lower classes would be chosen, either one who had more milk than her own child required or whose breasts were still engorged following the loss of an infant. The book of Exodus in the Old Testament relates how Moses' sister asked Pharaoh's daughter: 'Shall I go and call thee a nurse of the Hebrew women to nurse ye the child?'

When nursing has these traditional associations with femininity it is scarcely surprising that, in the eyes of most people, the male nurse is still something of an anomaly. Nursing is one sphere of human activity in which it is generally regarded as a positive advantage to be a woman, and the public image of the nurse is of a figure with distinctly female outlines. When a nurse is primarily thought of as a substitute mother or sister, ascribed roles (sex) and roles which have been achieved through training ideally merge in the same individual, it then seems odd when the person who has learned to be a nurse turns out to be a brother, or simply a helpful male. Male nurses tend to congregate in male psychiatric and geriatric wards, where the outward emphasis is on physical strength and their appearance in other spheres of nursing, such as health visiting, for example, is still rather exceptional. Women doctors, in our culture, are liable to suffer from a corresponding discrepancy between their public image and their personal identity.

Earliest nurses

However, there are indications that the very earliest hospital nurses may have been men. From ancient India, Sanscrit records supply accounts of a highly developed system of medicine and surgery which included the establishment of hospitals. The Indian hospitals may have been the first examples of state medicine, staffed by doctors and nurses paid by the government. It is difficult to put a precise date to these historic fore-runners of our present

48

system, but it might have been as long ago as 1600 B.C. Like our own contemporaries, the authorities of those days were preoccupied with the ideal attributes of the nurse. They wanted skill and reliability combined with a readiness to do anything which the patient's condition required. The fact that the attendants were all men may have related to the inferior position of women in that society.

In the worship of Aesculapius the Romans probably made some provision for the sick, but we have no knowledge of the people who were involved in the reception of the patients or worshippers at the temple associated with the Aesculapian cult.

It was Christianity which specifically enjoined the care of the sick and suffering as a duty upon the faithful and a means whereby they could gain grace, so the late Roman Empire and the mediaeval period witnessed a great expansion of religious institutions in which the piety of the worshippers and the needs of patients could happily meet. A variety of establishments were set up, where nuns and monks cared for the needs of all manner of unfortunates, travellers and the poor being accommodated as well as the sick. A hospital attached to a monastery in Constantinople in the twelfth century is known to have numbered women physicians among its female staff. The medical historian, Rosen, considers that these women, working only in the female ward, may well have been what we would term skilled midwives.

The Moslems, who contributed notably to early surgical techniques, had a hospital in Baghdad one thousand years ago. Not long afterwards, the description of a hospital in Cairo specifically mentioned both male and female nurses.

The first hospital in England was founded in York in A.D. 937. Like the others which soon followed, it was a multi-purpose religious institution to which people with all kinds of infirmities were admitted. Our own distinctions between physical and mental illness, and between poverty and the diseases associated with poverty had not been

49

made and the early hospitals were primarily refuges for the poor and needy. Whereas it would be difficult to conceive of a hospital nowadays without a doctor, some of the early mediaeval hospitals did not include any physician in their staff. It is clear that they were much closer in conception and function to the old style mixed workhouses of Victorian days than to a modern hospital designed for the treatment of acutely ill patients. Another analogy might be with an old people's 'home' today, since in our society, it is most often the elderly who by reason of social and financial deprivation, require a common shelter provided by society to supply their basic needs. When considering the forerunners of the modern hospital, therefore, it is important to remember that they were essentially substitutes for a home and that the sort of service which they supplied was such as the members of a family would ordinarily provide for one another.

Nurse as servant

Beginning with the view of the nurse as a caring mother or sister we now begin to perceive another element in her composite picture, that of the servant, the provider of service. In recent times the idea of domestic service has come to seem humiliating and despicable and the person who performs tasks to do with removing the debris of other people's lives is currently accorded a very low status in society. But, when Christian ideals were first spreading throughout Europe, service to others was a religious duty and humble tasks were sometimes deliberately undertaken by the wealthy and privileged to improve their chances of salvation. Our contemporary culture sets very great store upon acquired skills and upon intelligence and, since many domestic activities require the minimum of expertise, they tend to be underrated.

Dangerous dirt

But there is another significant aspect to our feelings
about personal service and this has to do with ideas concerning dirt and danger. There is no doubt that the
maintainance of life requires people who can deal with all
manner of accumulated dirt. It is necessary to dispose of
excreta, to wash soiled garments, to scrape cold food
remnants off plates, to wipe mucus from running noses and
smeared faeces off buttocks, to clean up vomit and
menstrual blood. When the products of various bodily
functions are itemised we may feel something of the
elemental revulsion which they arouse in the majority of
mankind. It seems as though any substance which has once
been inside the human body is shunned, as though it carried
a unique capacity to harm or contaminate. Every culture
inculcates strict rules about these bodily functions and
instructs its young in the correct manner of dealing with
them. To be more precise, it is in fact the mothers who
first clean their own offspring and later teach them how
to do it for themselves. In relation primarily to their own
infants but also, by extension, to other small helpless human
beings, most women are able to avoid the disgust attendant
upon double incontinence and to wipe with tenderness all
the leaking orifices. Without such early intimate attentions,
the human species could not survive.

By the time children are six or seven, they are expected
to have fully learnt the correct behaviour in relation to
the disposal of different forms of dangerous dirt. They
should know how to 'keep themselves clean' and failure
to do so may be taken as a sign of mental retardation.
Similarly, dirty habits in adults, sometimes described as a
regression to childhood, may be associated with serious
mental illness.

Later on, with the arrival of puberty, society enforces
rules to do with menstruation, a mysterious female process

which men in many parts of the world have regarded with peculiar dread.

Wherever many people live together it is necessary for certain kinds of waste to be removed from the vicinity of domestic dwellings, for sewage to be dealt with and household garbage destroyed. Some societies, as in India, for example, designate a despised caste of menials to perform these objectionable tasks. In most advanced societies, developments in public sanitation have rendered such jobs progressively less unpleasant, but the people who are physically involved in them do occupy a low position on the social class scale. The dustman ranks beneath the sanitary inspector, for example.

In circumstances of normal health, personal hygiene is a simple matter; although habits vary according to upbringing and housing conditions, the healthy adult manages these matters unaided and alone. However, when illness incapacitates someone to the extent that he can no longer control or cope with his bodily functions, the need for some kind of help is imperative. But it is a form of aid peculiarly distasteful to most people and, as nursing has evolved, this sort of personal service has gradually been delegated to lower and lower ranks in the hierarchy: it is passed down to grades of staff occupying the very lowest status. By reducing physical contact with certain categories of human debris the nurse has tried to avoid the implied social pollution which is consequent upon its proximity.

A striking contrast between the modern nursing profession's attitude towards dirt and that of a very unusual community, namely the community of aspiring saints, is provided in the writings of St Theresa. She recounts how, in order to mortify her flesh in the most extreme manner possible, she would sometimes force herself to take into her mouth the sputum which beggars had spat out. This repellent action, which seems to us extraordinarily misguided and hazardous from the medical point of view, also demonstrates the extremes to which someone aiming at humble service could go.

Prestige levels of bodily service

But, forgetting such saintly excesses, it is only in a fairly elaborately developed system of hospital nursing that the complete delegation of lowly or lower grade tasks can be achieved. When this does occur, there is always the sneaking possibility that the lower grade of attendants may be removing an important element of nursing along with the slops. In private home nursing, in district nursing, and in hospitals where staff is short, one person may be obliged to encompass functions which are preferably avoided. Because the circumstances are in some way unusual, the nurse who is reduced to carrying out menial jobs does not risk losing caste. For example, although a nurse in a ward with a whole range of auxiliaries, attendants and domestics would not descend to sluicing bed pans, if she were a district nursing sister attending a solitary old patient she would not hesitate to empty the commode.

The fine distinctions which can be made between differed aspects of bodily attention to patients mean less to the recipient than to the attendant. While nurses may well wish to avoid 'dirty' work and distribute their duties according to skills, the patient may feel deep gratitude towards the person who helps him in these ways. Such feelings relate to a sense of returning to the complete dependency of early childhood. Once again, the image of the mother merges with that of the nurse and the service which is required and given may appear in a favourable light, rather than implying any inferiority in the helper.

When nursing was entirely an unskilled family affair these subdivisions in types of care were less in evidence, although, if the household were sufficiently well off, servants might deal with slops, laundry and cleaning, leaving gentler ministrations to the mother. The preparation of invalid diets and, if necessary, their personal administration to the patient, would tend to be the chosen responsibility of the wife or mother. Washing the patient's garments constituted a lowlier and less important task than washing the patient. Moreover, since bathing involves seeing and touching the private parts of a patient's body, it is socially more appropriate that it should be carried out by someone whose relationship permits such intimate relations. In poor families, of course, any delegation and grading of duties is difficult and the ablest female member has generally to provide all the necessary nursing services.

Nursing before Nightingale

Moving from the most menial type of service to other life supports which are required by someone in the role of patient, it is clear that there are further aspects of home-making or housekeeping involved. Patients need to be housed, clothed and fed and their requirements in these essential respects require to be supervised by a responsible person. Before the formal training of nurses had been intro-duced, the matron in a hospital was a mother in the sense that she had to ensure that the place was adequately furnished and staffed and the inmates clad and fed. The fact that standards of adequacy in regard to any of these items would be seriously questioned today is irrelevant. The point is that the matron was, originally, a keeper of things rather than people, she was there in the position of a quarter-master, housekeeper, or storekeeper, respon-sible to the Board of Management or the Governors for all the physical impedimenta of the hospital. She would engage the cook, and see that merchants delivered supplies of bread, meat and beer. Finally, she would look for suitable local women to serve as nurses.

The conditions which prevailed in the hospitals, poor-houses and infirmaries of this country up until a hundred years ago have been well and graphically described by

Abel-Smith and it would be neither possible nor appropriate to summarise his historical account. But his and many other records supply further elements in the complex, composite picture of the nurse and may help us to understand some of her present role conflicts. There is little doubt that the stereotype of the nurse in the pre-Nightingale era still influences her distant descendants, although most of them would wish to disclaim any generic connection with their discredited old grandmothers.

The nurses whom the matrons of those days employed were, for the most part, middle-aged or elderly women, rich in experience of life but short of means and so reduced to seeking employment in the wards. The work was hard and exceptionally unpleasant, the hours were long, the pay was poor, and food was either scarce or no part of the bargain. Furthermore, the patients were rough, dirty and uninhibited. Remember that it was only poor people who in these days were reduced to entering hospital, and that standards of hygiene were so low as to be laughable. After all, these were the days in which surgeons operated in their frockcoats.

In the constitution of many hospitals and infirmaries the duties of the nurse were summed up in words like these: 'To obey the matron as her mistress and to behave with tenderness to the patients and with civility and respect to strangers.' The actual tasks of the nurse amounted to little more than keeping the patients as comfortable as possible, changing beds, cleaning floors and taking bottles to and from the apothecary's shop. The nurse, who was often alone on a ward, had no training apart from what she picked up on the job and she was seldom entrusted with any specifically medical tasks. For example, the application and removal of dressings was often done by student dressers, who were doctors in training, and the same medical students might be expected to watch over critically-ill patients at night to ensure that they had proper attention, although sometimes special night 'watchers' would be temporarily employed for this purpose.

However, the working conditions of nurses in the voluntary hospitals, which had been built by public subscription for the care of the sick, were appreciably better than those of the nurses in the contemporary poorhouses. The poorhouses had been established (in Elizabethan times) as a form of indoor, parish relief for the destitute. The whole purpose of the Victorian workhouses or poorhouses was to discourage anyone from entering; the institutions were deliberately forbidding and bleak, near-starvation diets were served and there was much actual cruelty as well as sheer neglect. It came as a surprise to the public to discover that a sizeable proportion of the pauper inmates were also sick. This does not seem in the least strange to use now, as we have become used to the idea that poverty makes people more liable to illness and that illness brings financial hardships. But the workhouse governors were somewhat taken aback by the pressing necessity to make minimal provision for sick inmates. The workhouse infirmaries did, however, have a most convenient source of labour to hand, namely the paupers themselves. Some of the so-called 'able-bodied' pauper women therefore doubled as nurses for their fellow lodgers. A not too distant parallel could be drawn between this situation and that in the Nazi concentration camps, where certain prisoners were selected to act as nurses.

The old style, untrained nurse of the last century acquired a reputation for being dirty, disreputable and unreliable. In it for the money, the small beer, bribes and any favours that came her way, she was frequently drunk and not above jumping into bed with the male patients. She came from the same social class as the patients did, she shared their language and responded to their bawdy jokes. Irreligious and irreverent, she was far removed indeed from the holy sisters of the former church hospices. What most distinguished her from her predecessors and the nurses who were to replace her was her undoubted accessibility.

As Abel-Smith has pointed out, history hitherto may have done her an injustice, by drawing a caricature of a woman who could well have supplied a friendly and comforting presence. So long as medicine was not a science and no one knew about the importance of cleanliness, a nurse's technical capacities and moral standards meant and mattered less than her capacity for caring. Then, as now, there were undoubtedly considerable individual differences in the attitudes of nurses towards their patients; the evidence also suggests that different standards of behaviour and care prevailed from one hospital or infirmary to another.

To summarise the social divisions of nursing in the period prior to the introduction of formal training: at the very bottom were the pauper nurses, closely identified with the destitute workhouse inmates from whose ranks they had been recruited; slightly higher were the nurses in voluntary hospitals, who enjoyed marginally better pay and conditions, but whose circumstances were still insufficient to attract other than working class women; sisters, in charge of wards, who had seldom been nurses themselves and were frequently recruited from outside, comprised what might be termed respectable, lower middle class women; at the top were the matrons, of a much superior class to the others, with responsibility for administering and ordering the day-to-day management of the hospital. Thus the three main grades of female hospital occupations existed independently of one another, like separate rock strata, they came from different sources and were never expected to mix.

In the first chapter mention was made of the relatively simple society which existed in Britain before the advent of the industrial revolution and how industrialisation and new inventions brought increased specialisation of jobs in more complex organisations, so that individuals came to play a multiplicity of social roles. Shortly, as a result of advances in medical science, a similar revolution was to begin in nursing and hospital administration, resulting eventually in a highly complicated hierarchical structure. This new organisation was to be very different from the former hospital arrangements modelled upon the domestic scene, where nurses who were part chars and part mother substitutes performed their simple duties.

Medical and social change

The Victorian era was a time of great social and legislative change and rapid scientific developments. Some of the most significant took place in the field of medicine, having to do with the discovery of the bacterial origin of many diseases, with the associated development of antiseptic and aseptic techniques, and the discovery of anaesthesia. Surgical methods were improved and extended and a whole variety of instruments and laboratory investigations rendered the diagnosis and treatment of disease considerably more precise and scientific than had been the case previously. There was still a long way to go before the pharmacological revolution of our own times and acute infections were still very common, but hospital medicine had taken on a more positive aspect and direct intervention in many disease processes was possible.

The progress in patient care was paralleled by developments in public health, the importance of pure water supplies and adequate sanitation were realised during this period and tangibly expressed in terms of civic sanitary engineering. Standards of living generally improved, especially as far as the middle and upper classes were concerned, and more money brought better housing, better diet and better hygiene.

Women from the poorer classes in Britain had always been accustomed to working very hard. In the pre-industrial days they had well defined areas of responsibility in household management and in work on the land in addition to

58

their primary concerns of bearing and rearing children. When large numbers of people moved into the new towns women had to take up very poorly paid employment either in their own homes or outside in factories, mills and mines where, often accompanied by their small children, they engaged in a desperate, daily struggle to maintain the family viability. The women who went to work in hospitals in those days were, in effect, part of the vast army of domestic servants.

However, at the same time as entire families in poverty could barely keep alive by their combined labours, the middle class were enjoying a period of unparalleled affluence and expansion. Unmarried ladies from well-to-do households were relieved of domestic chores and, possessed of a superior education and a Christian urge to service, they found it difficult to use their surplus energies or usefully express their altruism. Whereas their married sisters were fully occupied with family duties, most spinsters led lives of boredom and enforced idleness, prevented by strict social restraints from practically any form of paid employment.

Objectives of new nurse training

When Florence Nightingale, recently returned from her nursing and administrative triumphs in the Crimea, determined to institute a systematic training for nurses she was proposing reforms for which society was already partly prepared. Medicine now demanded a higher standard of nursing and a higher standard of nursing recruits were ready and waiting in the wings, eager to perform upon a stage which Miss Nightingale had lately sanctified by her presence.

In laying down the lines which the novices in nursing must follow, she was influenced by three main considerations. First, she was aware of the difference which good nursing care could make to the patients' well-being; second, she knew that the doctor's primary requirement was for reliability in the performance of their nursing assistance; third, she realised that the potential nurses needed the reassurance of a totally new image before they would venture into the wards.

The details of the introduction of training schemes and the mixed reception they first encountered, whilst of considerable historical interest, are not immediately relevant here. It is, however, important to analyse the elements of the new roles which these fundamental changes introduced into nursing and to consider the changed image of the nurse which was now so carefully fostered in the public eye.

Up until this point it has been possible to contemplate nursing practically without reference to doctors. By the middle of the last century, however, the physician had made his powerful influence felt upon the hospital scene and his effect upon the nurses' functions and their organisation became increasingly important. By this time the hospital specialist held a high position in society and there was widespread respect for his specialised skills. It was no longer possible or practicable for doctors to carry out all treatments themselves. The primary function of the physician was in the examination of patients in order to decide whether they were ill, whether they could be allowed to adopt the sick role. Having decided this, the physician had next to diagnose the nature of the illness before finally proceeding to prescribe treatment. The economical use of the doctor's skills and time, allowing him to diagnose and prescribe for the maximum number of patients required that he should be able to rely upon someone else to set the treatment in motion. Moreover, since the doctor could only spend a short time with each case and since it was important that he should be kept informed as to the results of treatment, someone must be available to watch the patient's progress closely and to report to him on his next visit about how things were going.

When treatment was largely non-specific and symptomatic it required the minimum of skill in its application. The various medicines, poultices, pills, ointments and paints may have brought relief but, with few exceptions, the patient's own powers of resistance were the dominant factors in recovery. Supportive measures, like special foods, stimulants in the form of wines and spirits, and the local application of heat and massage, were all procedures which were relatively easy to carry out and which necessitated neither precision nor regularity. Similarly, assessment of the patient was for long a matter of the unaided use of the senses, observing a flush, a sweat or a change of colour, placing a cool hand upon a fevered brow, noticing if the stools were unusual or if the urine was dark or tasted sweet.

But, as methods of diagnosis, forms of treatment and the means of assessment were all increasingly refined, as medicine became more scientific and efficient, the necessity arose for a very much higher standard of ward nursing than had formerly been supplied by one elderly maid of all work.

Need for specialisation in hospital

In the hospital, as in the industrial world outside its walls, specialisation meant that many more people would hitherto be required to carry out separate aspects of the total care of patients. Each person would be given a specific role to play in the larger organisation and it was vital that they could be relied upon to carry out their duties with precision and with a proper sense of personal responsibility.

It is useful to make the analogy with military service where, since the overriding aim is to defeat a known enemy, every member of the force must be prepared to give unquestioning obedience to their superior officers. A strict hierarchy is established so that the orders of the colonel-in-chief can be transmitted downwards, through all the succeeding regimental ranks. Indeed, these military ideals were clearly in the minds of the originators of the new system of nursing training, derived from Miss Nightingale's experiences with the armed forces and also from the example of a German nursing school in Kaiserwerth. In the battle against disease and death which had now for the first time been seriously joined, hospital discipline required to be of a similar nature and order to that which obtained on a fighting field.

Means of enhancing group loyalty

It has long been appreciated that certain techniques are especially effective for inducing a group of separate people to act together as one unit and become identified with the aims of a large organisation. For example, religious orders have always insisted that novices who join their ranks should begin by discarding most of their individual attributes. Leaving their old, worldly garments behind, they put on a new habit or uniform. The uniformity of appearance at once symbolises and contributes to a new sense of group identity and new habits of mind. Those in training live together, separated from the world they have left. They follow a strict routine, they may share physical deprivations and personal freedom is usually severely curtailed. This applies to all kinds of 'total institutions', to use the phrase of the sociologist, Goffman, meaning places where, for one reason or another, a new style of life is being deliberately imprinted and imposed and where every aspect of life takes place within the institution. The members of such a group begin before long to think of themselves as having a unique importance and purpose. The individual members change their reference group from former family and friends to the new group of which they now form humble units. Their main concern comes to be the regard and esteem of their peers and their superiors.

New standards, new values, new ideals become their own and it is hoped that they will shortly acquire a sense of regimental pride or a feeling of found affiliation with the aims of their order.

The process of training which the new recruits to nursing underwent in the middle of the last century could not have been better designed to produce a disciplined corps of female workers with a strong sense of professional identity. The probationers had to live in, under close supervision, so that their private lives became strictly subservient to their public duty. The three-year course was hard, but the ultimate rewards for those who could endure it were considerable, in the form of rapid promotion to sister or matron within hospitals or lucrative private practice without.

New professional image

The image of the new style nurse was intended as a complete contrast to that of her casual, amateurish predecessor. In place of a sluttish, amiable female of dubious morals, the Nightingale model appeared as a fresh young girl, pure in body and mind. She was 'sober, steadfast and demure', and represented an ideal of piety and personal service to which any daughter of a respectable middle-class family might aspire. With impeccable morals she combined skilled powers of observation, technical competence and a reliability which sprang from the habit of implicit obedience.

Nursing hierarchy

It is no wonder that this transformation pleased the patients, the public and the parents of probationers. On the part of some doctors, however, who stood to benefit greatly from the enhanced efficiency of their new assistants, there were certain reservations, since they perceived in this

63

beautiful female metamorphosis a hidden threat to their former unquestioned authority. Although the new, trained nurse was undoubtedly superior to her predecessors in terms of patient care and although the discipline she had learned to accept derived ostensibly from the orders of doctors regarding the treatment of patients, it was clear that a rival hierarchy was in process of rapid formation, a status system whose members owed ultimate allegiance not to the doctors but to the matron. Some physicians definitely preferred a situation in which they could directly command the services of a domestic to the new arrangements which necessitated their communicating with a trained nurse or sister, who then proceeded to delegate and divide the treatment tasks according to her own discretion, passing the orders down her own line of command.

Undoubtedly the matrons and their subordinates stood to gain enormously, in terms of power and prestige, from this new system. Although their duties were still administrative, the new matrons or lady superintendents now stood at the apex of a professional pyramid, made up by the several ranks of sisters, nurses, assistant nurses and probationers. No longer were they merely housekeepers; they kept the whole nursing staff under their supreme jurisdiction, simultaneously presenting a formidable challenge to their male, medical counterparts.

The process which has just been described, resulting in the establishment of a much more complex organisation of labour within the hospital and allowing the emergence of a distinct new group, with its own identity and group loyalties, has since been repeated many times within the broad field of health and welfare. Its implications are worth serious consideration, since they provide clues to the understanding of conflicts between different sections of the health professions and also because the process has important repercussions for the one group whom all the others are theoretically designed to serve, namely the patients.

For example, as other paramedical specialities have emerged, like physiotherapy and radiology, separate hospital departments have been established to which their employees, in the form of physiotherapists, radiographers and so on, give their first allegiance. Similarly, specialisation has meant that hospital domestic work (however defined) becomes the responsibility of a domestic supervisor. Meanwhile, outside hospitals altogether, there are branches of community nursing, such as health visiting, whose members have a sense of identity which they may be particularly anxious to maintain and foster when another paramedical group of would-be professionals, the social workers, appears over the horizon. The establishment of distinctive groups, with limited functions and responsibilities, clarifies the roles which their individual members have to fulfil. They convey a comforting sense of security and permanence which is increased by ritual occasions when members meet to reiterate what they have in common and how they differ from all the others who are 'outsiders'.

Another way of looking at this process is to regard it as a form of adult socialisation, a learning experience which results in a change of outlook on the part of the individual, who thereafter views the world in a new light. This is obviously the case with the kind of training involved in a profession like nursing or medicine, at the end of which the individual has acquired entirely new habits of thought, couched in a new language.

Advantages and drawbacks

Now, in a great many respects, the special view and the unique identity which result from a process of training in an exclusive group or school is valuable. It means that all those who have been through the course and have become accepted members of the group can communicate quickly and easily, they can take many assumptions for granted,

65

they use terms familiar to one another, all of which simplifies the jobs upon which they are mutually engaged. They know, for example, who takes precedence, whom they must obey and to whom they may issue commands or offer authoritative advice. But the complexity of the organisation to which they all belong and their total involvement in this group may, at the same time, tend to reduce their appreciation of those who stand outside it. This may not matter much if the outsiders are people whom they rarely encounter, but it does matter a great deal if the outsiders are the very clients whom the organisation has been set up to serve. Hence the paradox that makes the increased complexity and specialisation of nursing (or medicine) a possible source of conflict with the patient's interests. The more the nurse sees her first responsibility as being to the ward sister, the matron, the training school or her colleagues, the more liable she may be to forget the patient's point of view. The more she knows of the specialised language of nursing and medicine the greater the danger that a diagnostic label may effectively conceal from her the individual patient and his pressing personal anxieties.

However, at the time when a comprehensive, three-year scheme of training was first introduced in nursing, any incidental disadvantages of increased professionalism were far outweighed by its obvious merits, and it was hoped that eventually all hospitals would be entirely staffed by nurses who were trained or in training.

Characteristics of a profession

Since much of this chapter has been concerned with the search for professional identity, a word is appropriate regarding some of the distinguishing characteristics of a profession. The members of a profession have had, firstly, to undertake a prolonged and severe period of training; following this, they are faced with some kind of trial or test, what the anthropologists would term a 'rite of passage'; if they pass this formal test they must then give tacit agreement to certain moral precepts which will govern their subsequent behaviour; finally, they are ritually admitted to the ranks of the profession, a process which often involves the addition of their names to an exclusive register or roll and the conferring of documents which give tangible evidence of their symbolic acceptance.

In the case of nursing, the Royal College of Nursing laid down the course of training and the final tests whilst the General Nursing Council held the solemn register to which aspiring professionals were ultimately to be admitted, and the aim of these two powerful proponents of the nurse's unique role was to limit the epithet 'nurse' to those who had successfully navigated the straight and narrow path to registration. The midwives, meanwhile, developed independently along parallel lines. But, from the very first time when a conscious effort was made to elevate, refine and restrict the concept of nursing and midwifery until the present day, these attempts at exclusiveness have tended to be frustrated by the sheer extent of human need and the multiplicity of modes of caring. If the dividing line between nurses and non-nurses is set too high there will be continual difficulties in providing complete care of the patient. Nursing activities have undoubtedly been undertaken by human beings for one another since the dawn of time and will continue into the unforeseeable future, whatever names are given to those who offer support. So if 'nurses' decide that certain areas of activity are inappropriate for them it does not dispose of the problem, which then becomes a matter of discovering (and training) new categories of 'carers' or helpers who are prepared to cope.

The specialisation in medicine which commenced in the last century has gained considerable momentum over the past twenty-five years. Diagnostic and therapeutic skills have become highly developed in all the separate branches of the discipline, in obstetrics, in neo-natal paediatrics, in orthopaedics, in anaesthesia, in cardiac intensive care and in transplant surgery, to name only a few. At the same time, the phenomenal increase in the range of effective drugs which are available have made possible the control of formerly fatal infections and the amelioration, if not the cure, of all manner of common ills. The high cost of modern hospital care for acute conditions has forced a changing pace of work in the wards, since it is essential that expensive beds and resources should not be wasted, there is a pressure for shorter stays in hospital and patients are soon sent back into the community. All these developments demand a hitherto unprecedented level of professional efficiency on the part of nurses, both inside and outside hospital.

Recent concern with management

It is therefore not surprising that there should have been much concern in Britain lately with management skills in nursing. As a member of a hierarchical structure, responsible for organising the complex activities of many others, the trained nurse undoubtedly needs organisational ability. She also deserves the incentives which a clear career ladder in higher management affords. There is, however, a danger that concentration on the status system and its detailed operation can become disproportionate, deflecting attention from the special objectives and tasks with which nursing, as a unique human occupation, is concerned.

Patient's needs

But there are already countervailing tendencies at work. This is evidenced by a publication like the Briggs Report which, with eloquence and scholarship, has sought to create a new image for nursing in the latter part of the twentieth century. The leaders of nursing are now endeavouring to re-orientate the profession in the direction of patients' needs. They have started with a realistic appraisal of the wide variety of nursing services which people now require, both in the community and in all kinds of hospital settings, from short stay units to institutions for prolonged care. They have emphasised that the rate of change which the profession have hitherto experienced is likely to continue or even accelerate, so that nurses must be infinitely adaptable if they are to cope with future demands and provide any degree of continuity of care for patients who are liable to move swiftly from home to hospital and back again.

The Briggs Committee has very logically gone on to propose changes in basic nurse training to bring about the aims which they see are necessary. The old barriers between separate sections of our health service are in process of being broken down but the people who work in the service need to change their attitudes if administrative rearrangements are to have any real meaning for the public. Clearly, the best place to start is with the new recruits, in this case among nurses in training.

There are many excellent reasons for divisions of labour in medicine and for clear lines of authority, but much medical care in the future will depend for its success on the ability of the members of different caring professions to work together, in teams. This is no easy or automatic matter, because once people have grown to accept divisions changes may cause alarm and a sense of insecurity. In a later chapter we shall revert to this theme and consider some of the ways in which nurses are already changing their modes of working to adapt to new needs and circumstances

But let us return finally to the patient's point of view on nursing, the view of the outsider. In a sense, the nurse has had to be all things to all men. Thus, she includes in her image the outline of the nurse as nun, virginal and untouchable, yet possessing a gentle, sisterly touch. Many nurses have in the past been nuns, but not all nurses evoke this picture or appear in such a pure guise in their patients' phantasies, for the nurse can also arouse desire and is a popular figure in fictional romance. Furthermore, many nurses nowadays are already married and, since the rest have a high statistical probability of marrying, the spinster domination of the profession is over. At the same time the nurse represents for the patient a uniformed member of the hospital establishment, entitled to command people older and wiser than herself by virtue of her association with the revered processes of healing. She is a very important intermediary between the anxious patient and the powerful doctor, able to interpret his decisions and intentions in simple terms and dispel some of the awe which surrounds his mysterious activities. However, compared to most patients she herself seems a very knowledgeable technical expert and patients can entertain great expectations of the most junior probationer. In some cases, and not only in mental hospitals, the nurse may appear to her charges in a custodial guise, restricting freedom and imposing seemingly arbitrary rules. To a patient in hospital the nurse is also in part a hostess, to whom polite gratitude is due. A few patients may realise that nurses can be teachers or students or managers. But to many, her primary attributes are motherly ones, compassion and caring and the capacity to relieve suffering, by whatever means.

Questions

1 Where do we first find some early written references to nurses?
  Were these nurses men or women and how were their duties defined?
2 What kind of inmates did the earliest European hospitals contain and how much resemblance did these hospitals bear to these of today?
3 Describe the women who were recruited to nursing in Britain in the 'pre-Nightingale' era.
4 What were the main objectives which Florence Nightingale

sought to achieve by her original system of nursing training?

5 Outline some of the ways in which a profession like nursing can develop a clear sense of identity and change the ways of thinking and behaving of its young recruits.

6 What does the phrase 'patient-orientated' mean to you?

7 Members of the public may have a different image of nursing from that of the profession.

  a How can you become aware of these differences?

  b How could such differences matter in practice?

Further reading

ABEL-SMITH, BRIAN (1960) *A History of the Nursing Profession,* Heinemann, London.

BROWN, ESTHER LUCILE (1966) 'Nursing and patient care', in *Sociological Essays,* ed. Fred Davis, John Wiley, New York.

MCFARLANE, JEAN K. (1970) *The Proper Study of the Nurse: The Study of Nursing Care,* Royal College of Nursing and National Council of Nurses, RCN, London.

PRATT, HENRY (1965) 'The doctor's view of the changing nurse-physician relationship', *Journal of Medical Education, 40,* 767-71.

RAMSDEN, GERTRUDE A. and SKEET, MURIEL H. (1967) *Marriage and Nursing,* Fifth Report of the Dan Mason Nursing Research Committee, London.

ROSEN, JUANITA and JONES, KATHLEEN (1972) 'The male nurse', in *Problems and Progress in Medical Care,* 7th series, Nuffield Provincial Hospitals Trust, Oxford University Press, London.

SCHLOTFELDT, ROZELLA M. (1965) 'The nurse's view of the changing nurse-physician relationship', *Journal of Medical Education, 40,* 772-7.

SEYMER, LUCY RIDGELY (1956) *A General History of Nursing,* Faber & Faber, London.

SHYROCK, RICHARD H. (1959) *The History of Nursing: An Interpretation of the Social and Medical Factors Involved,* W. B. Saunders, Philadelphia and London.

Reports

Senior Nursing Staff Structure (1966) (Salmon Committee Report), Ministry of Health and Scottish Home and Health Department, HMSO, London.

Relieving Nurses of Non-Nursing Duties in General and Maternity Hospitals (1968), Dept of Health and Social Security, Central Health Services Council, Report by the Sub-Committee of the Standing Nursing Advisory Committee, HMSO, London.

The Evaluation of Nursing Education (1969), Report of a Working Group, WHO Regional Office for Europe, Copenhagen.

The State Enrolled Nurse (1971), Dept of Health and Social Security, Central Health Services Council, Report by a Sub-Committee of the Standing Nursing Advisory Committee, HMSO, London.

Report of the Committee on Nursing (1972) Cmnd 5115, Chairman, Asa Briggs, HMSO, London.

IV The doctor in society

The doctor in previous cultures; Hippocrates and medical ethics; basis for doctors' authority; risk of abuse of trust; some contemporary problems for medical ethics; development of modern medicine from arts of surgery, medicine and the apothecaries; the process of medical education; medical auxiliaries, 'feldschers' and others; inter-professional strains and rivalries; the general practitioner's past and future; health centre organisation; the demystification of medicine.

In many previous cultures the healer was credited with heroic and divine attributes; he combined the roles of doctor and priest and his prophecies and prognoses were sought by men in search of fortunes, rulers proposing war or nations facing famine. Armed with the ability to intervene between mortal men and the mysterious forces which perpetually threaten their plans and their very existence, the doctor occupies a unique position of respect, since he is needed both by suffering individuals and by society at large. Severe illness, descending suddenly and unsought, constitutes a threat to the person and to the social group of which he forms a part; it emphasises men's essential vulnerability, causing them to seek both explanation and relief. To people or communities confronted by disease and possible disruption the doctor has offered means of placating fate and diverting misfortune. In his capacity as an expert in divination or diagnoses he has perceived the action best calculated to please the gods, appease the ancestors, combat the germs, or unravel psychic tensions, according to whatever happens to be the current view of sickness causation. He has named the unnamed terrors, thereby rendering them more manageable and less dreadful. At the same time the physician has provided ordinary patients and their families with the incalculable benefit which comes from casting the burden of illness and its attendant anxiety upon someone who is both wise and powerful. This chapter will trace some of the changes which have occurred in the doctor's position and functions in society, from early times until the present.

Even today, the most revered type of practitioner in certain traditional societies in other parts of the world is the one who can deal in magic and interpret the workings of fate. He studies his patients in their social setting, surrounded by people who may wish them ill, as well as by loved and loving relatives, and he tries to discern the personal discords which can contribute to their continued illness and mental disquiet. There are all kinds of divination procedures still current in Africa, for example, involving casting nuts and knuckle bones upon the ground, contemplating the fall of seed pods or the death throes of sacrificial chickens, from which chance happenings the priestly healer seeks to derive indications of his patient's past experience and prescribe his appropriate future action.

The doctor in other cultures

In ancient Greece, the followers of the God Aesculapius revered his memory in sacred shrines which attracted pilgrims eager to participate in the complex divination processes and healing rituals associated with his cult. This aspect of Greek medicine was closely bound up with religion, and the remedies which were dispensed had a predominantly supernatural or magical content. Similarly, in Egypt, the cult of Imhotep exemplified the same union of medicine and religion and demanded from sick suppliants a similar amalgam of faith and hope.

We who live in a period when medicine is supposed to be scientific may wonder how medical systems and practi-

74

tioners based upon such foolish superstitions ever managed to survive. How could people respect doctors who were magicians or place their confidence in spilt blood or scattered kola nuts? There are a number of reasons for the public faith in doctors, of every variety and historical period, and some of these reasons are totally unrelated to the proven efficacy of specific kinds of treatment. First, it is the case that most illnesses are not fatal, most patients do recover, whatever the therapy and, if they have been following a particular regime, they will probably attribute a favourable outcome to the procedures they have undergone on the instructions of whatever priests or practitioners they have consulted. In the second place, every anxiety requires some relief, and patronage of the local healer, credited with exceptional wisdom and skill, will in itself help to reassure someone who can no longer help himself. Finally, by making use of such expert advice as is available, the sick person and his relatives are acting in a socially acceptable fashion, they are participating in a form of social behaviour which they have learnt in childhood and which their own subsequent experience reinforces, they are seeking the services of someone who is officially deputed by society the responsibility of sanctioning the sick status, allowing the sick person to be excused from his obligations until such time as his present misfortune is past.

It would, however, be totally misleading to suggest that the physician or doctor has always enjoyed an aura of divinity. While some doctors or branches of medicine may have been associated with religious practices and fundamental anxieties, a great deal of illness and its care has belonged to a much more mundane level of experience. People with symptoms have always been in the habit of procuring simple remedies composed of ingredients close to hand to treat the many minor ailments which are inconvenient or uncomfortable rather than constituting any serious threat to life. The basis of this kind of medicine

75

is naturalistic and empirical, it takes into account the observable effect of various medicinal substances or physical procedures upon the course of individual illness. It builds up a core of knowledge and beliefs, consisting of specific prescriptions and items of practical advice related to diet and fresh air and exercise, the importance of regular excretory processes and the avoidance of sexual or alcoholic excesses. Thus, whilst certain categories of patients in ancient Greece might be visiting the shrine of Aesculapius, others would simply patronise a physician who was peddling his advice and wares in the open market place and who had more in common with a packman than a priest. Such doctors had to be observant, astute and quick thinking, being concerned to sell as many remedies as the local market would bear before moving on to a fresh pitch. A credible comparison can be drawn between their kind of medical practice and that of the herbalists who are even now the first source of advice for many sick people in under-doctored areas of the tropics. However, they must have included among their numbers unscrupulous 'quacks' who profited from people's credulity and made a dubious living from the misfortunes of their fellow men.

Hippocrates and medical ethics

Hippocrates is rightly revered as the founder of modern medicine. The texts connected with his name were probably collected in Greece about 400 B.C. and they are still remarkable for their detailed and arresting descriptions of the symptoms and signs of illness, the reasonable tone of their prescriptions and the good sense of the hygienic measures advocated for the prevention of disease and the promotion of good health. Being based upon careful physical observation, the Hippocratic writings represent a truly scientific approach to the problems of sickness. However, these early physicians did not light upon the idea of specific disease entities, they reported carefully upon the patient's general state, but they failed to discern behind the individual picture the manifestations of a definable illness. It is possible to draw a parallel between their practice and an important aspect of the work of a skilled nurse today who is properly less concerned with diagnoses than with noting the exact, measurable condition of her patients from hour to hour and day to day. It should be remembered that, at the time when the condition was first introduced, there were no instruments available to assist the medical attendant who had to depend upon his unaided senses to perceive all the subtle physical signs from which a favourable or fatal outcome might be foretold.

Modern medicine and nursing are both indebted to the Hippocratic Greek doctors in another important respect, the definition of medical ethics. In their writings they made explicit the obligations which a doctor must fulfil towards his patient as a corollary to the privileges afforded to a physician. In the interests of restoring health, the doctor is allowed unrestricted access to the bodies and minds of others and it is, therefore, essential that he should not abuse the reliance which patients place upon him. This is all the more necessary since the patient enters into an intimate relationship with his doctor at a time when illness and distress have rendered him peculiarly vulnerable and defenceless, so that nothing but the mutual expectation of morality can protect him. It must be accepted by both doctors and patients that the complementary roles which they are playing are guided by clear rules, each knowing what he may expect of the other.

Doctors still swear allegiance to some variant of the 'Hippocratic Oath' as part of the process of graduation, undertaking, for example, 'To practise the art of Medicine with care, with purity of conduct and with uprightness, faithfully attending to everything conducive to the welfare of the sick. ... Whatever things seen or heard in the course of medical practice ought not to be spoken of, I will not, save for weighty reasons, divulge.' A solemn public statement of this kind, summarising the ethics of intending practitioners, is one characteristic of a profession. Any group of people who are primarily involved in a vital service to the rest of society are accorded high status and special privileges. To constitute a profession rather than a mere association of similarly occupied individuals, the members need to share a lengthy and rigorous training. On its completion they vow allegiance to the ideal of the group in terms which establish both their identity with the group itself and their responsibilities outside it. Thereafter, they are largely subject to rules laid down by a governing body of their peers, which watches over their conduct and is empowered to take action to expel them from the profession should they fail, in some important respect, to conform.

Basis for doctor's authority

Before turning to the development of the different branches of medicine and surgery which preceded and influenced present day practice, it is appropriate to pause and summarise what constitutes the distinctive elements of the doctor's authoritative position in society. One sociologist (Paterson) has suggested the use of the term 'Aesculapian authority' for the combination of charisma, wisdom and morals which characterise the profession.

The word 'charisma' was coined by the nineteenth-century sociologist Weber. It refers to that quality of leadership which relates to non-rational motives, the quality which inspires faith by reason of its holder's association with supernatural powers and with matters of life and death. This is what we have been describing in the beginning of this chapter, to do with the doctor's role as a priestly mediator between men and fate. Doctors need not be entirely reasonable, and the most famous of them have often been admired for their eccentricity. Since life itself is uncertain and the workings of fate are strange, the doctor as magician mirrors the inconsistencies of human experience, meeting mystery with mystery.

However, added to this, the doctor earns respect because of his superior knowledge, gained in the course of a long apprenticeship and based upon his own experience and that of his seniors. This has been called 'sapiential authority', the right to be heard by reason of knowledge or expertise. Because they know more than their patients, doctors are qualified to advise them to take treatment in their own best interests. Nowadays this technical aspect of medicine has become much more prominent as medical and scientific discoveries have added enormously to useful knowledge.

Finally, the doctor is permitted to control and direct others because of his moral authority. Much of this moral authority is taken for granted by those who share the same culture with him, but it finds expression in statements such as the Hippocratic Oath which make it clear that whatever he does must always be primarily for the good of his patients. It is because the enterprise in which the doctor is engaged is essentially good and right, both for society and for the individual, that he is accorded moral authority as well as being revered for his knowledge and his powers over life and death.

Public expectations

This expression of the doctor's position is something of an oversimplification, since there are doctors who are much less engaged than others in intimate personal contact with patients and there are also some very difficult situations in which a doctor's duty to his patient may conflict with his duty to society. But the foregoing represents the essence of the public expectations of the profession, what is demanded of doctors, not necessarily as individuals, but by virtue of having achieved the public position of the physician. People think of doctors as being wise and powerful and they confidently expect them to behave well. The fact that all doctors do not come up to expectations is not the point; the behaviour of errant members is always being compared with an ideal.

Patients frequently persist in their faith in spite of depressing evidence that doctors have not conformed to a standard and people may be astonishingly lenient towards doctor's failings. This is partly because lay people cannot afford to distrust someone who occupies a position of power and influence in matters of literally vital importance. The very sick patient would feel utterly destitute if he allowed doubts to intervene. The extent of the public trust in them should imbue doctors with an increased sense of personal responsibility. If this is not the case, however, and the doctor is clearly failing to live up to the professional ideal, he is liable to be sanctioned by being 'struck off the register'. But patients do have legitimate complaints falling short of gross negligence and they often find it difficult to secure a hearing.

Doctors' political power

The unique respect accorded to the profession, and which they come to expect as a right, can also serve to inflate their self-importance and to emphasise intra-professional solidarity at the expense of the public. Just as the individual doctor has considerable influence over his patients at crisis points in their lives, so the profession as a whole has the power to affect policies relating to the health of an entire nation. This influence is seldom conveyed by crude threats of withdrawing labour, since to strike would itself undermine the altruistic basis for the profession's moral position, but pressure is constantly exerted by virtue of doctors' supposedly superior knowledge upon all kinds of matters relating to health. The doctors form an extremely powerful pressure group which no politician can afford to disregard.

There is no doubt that doctors generally try to reinforce

the favourable image of themselves as invariably hard-working, self-sacrificing, public-spirited people and that they tend to react unfavourably to criticism of their working hours and methods. Doctors need to be free to exercise their professional judgment in regard to patients' treatment, but this freedom should never be allowed to become neglect, on the one hand, or extravagant prescription on the other. The question of society's control over doctors is a delicate one and it is not easily resolved. But, since there are not unlimited financial resources for health and welfare, policy decisions do have to be taken at a high level which effectively determine the amount of money available, for example, for preventive or caring medicine as opposed to curative medicine. At another level, doctors may be restricted in the use of particularly expensive drugs; or they may be encouraged, by various incentives, to expand general practice facilities.

Even if the profession as a whole or individual members of it may sometimes fall short of the central ideals of service, confidentiality and respect for human life, it is still important that these ideals should continue to be respected. Society has a continuing stake in the ethical precepts which were formulated for physicians over two thousand years ago and which the profession has ever since avowed. The central position of doctors in the status system of a modern society is no accident since, both in their intentions and in their actions, they are concerned with the preservation of life and with respect for the individual person. Their function in maintaining the lives of patients and, by extension, the life of society as a whole, assures them of a powerful continuing influence.

Contemporary problems

As was mentioned earlier, the precise interpretation of the doctor's duty in many specific instances of con-temporary practice can be very difficult because of situations where the individual's welfare seems to conflict with that of the group to which he belongs. It is now possible to save the lives of babies who are born with severe congenital abnormalities. They would formerly have died very soon from infection but now this can be prevented and surgical manoeuvres can compensate for some of the physical disabilities. The presence of such a child will, of course, profoundly affect his family. Whom should the doctor mainly consider? Is he ever justified in withholding treatment or antibiotics from such babies or does his duty involve unwavering respect for human life? Similar dilemmas relate to the other extreme of life, since all kinds of techniques for prolonging life are now available. When should an old person be permitted to die 'naturally'? Transplant surgery has highlighted the necessity for a new definition of death; abortion can represent a conflict between the welfare of the unborn child and that of the mother; the restraint of patients whose behaviour is violent or unpredictable may be necessary to maintain family peace and public order. Then there is the question of whether people who have once been mentally ill should be encouraged to resume their previous occupation if it involves the care of young children. All of these are extremely difficult areas of decision making, in which the present guide lines are by no means clear and where different doctors may vary in the interpretation of their professional duty. But it is important that the public should continue to hold the view of the profession as being altruistic, dependable and humane.

Development of modern medicine

Although we tend to think of doctors as being part of a homogeneous professional group, which wields considerable power and can act to protect and further its members' own interests as well as those of patients, this unification and ordering of the profession has only come about gradually and within comparatively recent times. Formerly, there were three separate branches of medicine, the apothecaries, the physicians and the surgeons. Before the establishment of formal teaching in any of these areas, there was little in the way of licensing to limit the right to practise of anyone who felt he was competent to do so. In the Middle Ages surgeons were essentially craftsmen, usually combining surgery with barbering and the provision of bathing facilities. They eventually grouped themselves in guilds, like other artisans and, in this organisation, they were often conveniently joined with the blacksmiths who supplied their tools. Such a close association between barber surgeons and smiths persists to this day in Moslem communities in West Africa, which have derived their surgical traditions from the ancient world.

Physicians

The physicians occupied a more rarified field of ideas than did the surgeons and had undergone a liberal university education, which originally bore scant relationship to the facts of anatomy, physiology and pathology. As time went on, however, the curriculum of intending physicians became gradually longer, more relevant and more intensive examinations were introduced and, by the thirteenth century, European universities had begun to confer licences to practise. Some cities without a university set up their own colleges for the purpose of examining and authorising aspiring physicians; for example, the Royal College of Physicians in London (1518). The object of such licensing bodies was to limit the practice of medicine to those who were deemed fully qualified and to discourage the activities of numerous enterprising practitioners whose public claims to knowledge had never been put to an academic test.

Apothecaries

The apothecaries, who were the forerunners of our pharmacists, also formed themselves into guilds whose concerns, like those of the surgeons, were mainly practical. The early union in London of the apothecaries' guild with the grocers' guild indicated the common commercial interests of their members. King James I later granted their separation, on the grounds that the apothecaries really constituted a 'mystery' or proper profession, rather than a mere trade. Thereafter, the apothecaries began to train apprentices formally, teaching them the use of a number of effective drugs along with many strange concoctions which must have been based upon sympathetic magic. The apothecaries gradually extended their knowledge and practice, supplying the poor with a level of treatment and medication which they could not afford to purchase from expensive private physicians. In 1815, apothecaries were authorised to conduct private practice, but they were only allowed to charge for their medicine, so 'dosing' soon became synonomous with treatment. Physicians and surgeons continued to battle for supremacy for a long time and the apothecaries had to act as buffers between them, meanwhile collecting a sizeable clientele.

It was not until 1858 that an important Medical Act finally brought the three branches of medicine together, confining the legal right to practise to those whose names were enrolled upon the Medical Register. From this time onwards the profession had a common portal of entry, and any specialisation was subsequent to admission to the ordinary role of medical practitioner.

Medical education

The process of becoming a doctor in Britain today is a lengthy one, involving a period of five or six years' academic and clinical instruction followed by a further twelve month's work in hospital. The medical student graduates from his parent university after some six years, receiving a degree which signifies his successful completion of this part of the initiation process, but he is not accepted as being eligible to practise on his own until the subsequent year's apprenticeship has been completed. It is only then that he is 'registered' by the General Medical Council. Most of the ritual associated with the procedure attaches to graduation, an occasion of pomp and ceremony when the new graduate is publically acclaimed by family and former teachers as having achieved a totally new and significant status in society. For historical reasons, graduation has always been more momentous than registration; it is the time when an entire class passes through the same rites together, to the accompaniment of solemn pronouncements, vows and the repetitive recitation of names and distinctions.

Adult socialisation

However, the whole process of medical education can be regarded as another example of adult socialisation similar to that we described in the case of nursing. It profoundly alters the attitudes and outlook of a group of individuals and gradually makes them less and less like the laymen whom they once were and who will mainly comprise their future patients. In the seven or so years which the educational process takes, the intending doctor learns far more than facts; he learns a whole new view of the world, as his vision is trained to detect subtle signs of sickness in his fellows; he speaks and thinks in a new, medical language; he adopts new standards of behaviour; he accepts new values and comes to reverence new academic or professional heroes. Mundane experiences and appetites for food and drink, sex and cigarettes, take on a different meaning for him, since they are now perceived in a context which includes dangers and implications unknown to the ordinary layman. The long period that he has spent, in the company of others like him, absorbing strange, esoteric facts, mastering laboratory techniques, dissecting the bodies of the dead and labelling the ills of the living, eventually sets him apart, in a very important manner, from most of his fellows. This is, of course, the essence of professionalisation but, in addition to becoming learned in a particular sphere of human knowledge and proficient in an area which is important to society, the doctor has undergone special experiences which most other professions, apart from nursing, lack. He shares with them an intimate knowledge of suffering and death and he acquires unique respect by virtue of his ability to confront these awesome realities.

It is only slowly, as the young medical student proceeds through his course, that he acquires the charisma which attaches to the fully-fledged practitioner. Once he is allowed into the hospital wards, for instance, he will often be addressed by patients as 'Doctor' and this may not be simply because they fail to understand his junior status. He is regarded as almost a doctor. Nurses too, admire final year students more than their callow predecessors in the early years of medical school, being prepared to consider that they probably possess a lot of theoretical knowledge, although the nurses may be justifiably critical of the medical students' practical competence. Students who are still officially in the 'pre-clinical' part of their medical education may find considerable difficulty in participating in clinical case conferences, or even in addressing people labelled as 'patients', because of a feeling on the part of medical administrators and ward staff that such fledgling students are not yet properly 'medical' in any important sense. In other words, the privileges attached to the physician's role are not easily or suddenly acquired and most modern societies have tended to make it increasingly difficult for people to become doctors. Nevertheless, the notable rewards in terms of status, interest, power and money which accrue to the doctor's eventual position mean that there are always many more aspirants than places available.

Over the course of time, what a doctor needs to learn in order to function efficiently has tremendously increased, both in quantity and in complexity, so that one of the big current problems is what should be included in the crowded medical curriculum. There is a lot of debate, for instance, as to whether every new doctor should have gone through exactly the same basic undergraduate course or whether doctors in training should be allowed to develop special subject interests, with the inevitable corollary that they spend less time on something else. Does every doctor have to know about skin diseases or venereal disease, for example, or need he only know when to refer certain conditions to the appropriate specialists? Is there not a case for bringing doctors and nurses together at certain points of their training? Should they not have the experience of learning together if they are to work together?

Medical auxiliaries

In countries like our own, with a very heavy expenditure upon health and something like one doctor per two to three thousand of the population, the debate is over relatively minor changes in a very long training for the complete professional. But in many parts of the world the need for medical care is far in excess of the available trained doctors and the terms of the debate are rather different. Then the question of training a new sort of doctor arises. Some communist countries and also parts of Africa have favoured the development of a practitioner who has limited diagnostic skills and restricted treatment functions. Such auxiliaries are educated for a relatively brief period of time and they must confine their activities to simple medical situations, referring any cases with which they cannot cope to a fully-qualified practitioner. In communities which find it impossible to supply medical care in anything like the quantity or quality to which we are accustomed, this arrangement ensures at least a modicum of care for sick people who would otherwise completely lack modern forms of treatment and effective medicines.

Professional resistance

This is clearly a matter in which both doctors and nurses are intimately concerned, for the health worker in question is in some sense a hybrid, combining characteristics of both the nursing and the medical profession, and the last chapter will take a closer look at 'nurse practitioners'. As far as doctors are concerned, however, the idea of introducing a lower level operator has certainly not been universally popular, even in countries where patients' needs would seem to demand some such compromise. Those who have been through the protracted training necessary for qualification in the ordinary way are reluctant to grant the title of doctor to others who have avoided the painful process of initiation. Doctors also see possible difficulties in actual practice, where a 'feldscher' (see p. 152) might be tempted to take on more than his experience justified, thereby depriving the 'real' doctor of patients as well as doing actual harm. There seems to be an underlying fear of any reduction of the fully-qualified doctor's status by the addition of less highly-qualified practitioners with whom the public might confuse them. One might think that the community's need for some measure of trained care and attention should take precedence over the private anxieties of a professional pressure group. But this is an instance where the concerted opinion of a profession may act against any change which is perceived as threatening and doctors are usually in a position to exert powerful pressure upon those who formulate public policies.

In the developing countries of Africa the introduction of a new grade of doctor has often been resisted for a further reason; it is looked upon as a device to fob off a poor quality product upon poor nations. Countries which have fairly recently secured independence from the former colonial powers want to demonstrate that they are capable of achieving the same standards as the West in professional education and practice. Thus, the urge to establish medical schools represents a desire for a notable status symbol as well as a means of supplying patients with specialised care. There is the feeling that 'only the best is good enough' and suggestions for the training of medical auxiliaries are likely to be regarded as a neo-colonialist ruse, which must be resisted by self-respecting nationalists.

It is only fair to add that the reasons for the medical profession's reluctance in various countries to countenance new grades and types of health worker do not all relate to self-interest. Doctors wish to preserve a close relationship with individual patients whose personal welfare has always been the physician's prime concern. Doctors certainly tend to be conservative in outlook and view with suspicion innovations which may disturb clinical practice as they have always known it. This fundamental resistance to change means that they sometimes lag behind their patients and the rest of society and are surprised to discover new attitudes and expectations on the part of the public.

General practitioners

Many doctors take it for granted that they should occupy a pedestal from which to deliver unquestioned pronounce-ments and yet they complain about the 'unreasonable demands' which patients nowadays make of them. Doctors in general practice are especially liable to express dissatis-faction with their position, complaining about the burden of unremitting toil which they claim is their lot and the inadequate rewards which contemporary society gives them. Although their resentment is frequently phrased in financial terms, closer enquiry reveals fundamental anxieties about a diminution in public respect, a suspicion on the part of doctors that they no longer count for so much, either in the community or in the eyes of individual patients.

In part these professional fears and resentments have been associated with the provision of a national health service in Britain which, in effect, gives everyone the right to free medical treatment. In this system the general practitioner holds a key position, since he is the doctor whom patients must approach first and who decides whether referral to a specialist is necessary. But some general practitioners have resented the principle of free access upon which their own livelihood and position depends and object to the wide range of problems which patients continually bring to them for sorting out. Doctors who have been trained to diagnose and treat serious and rare illnesses under hospital conditions are often surprised to discover the triviality of most of the symptoms and ills which afflict their patients and they may feel impatient about the multiple, simple worries which cause people to seek a doctor's help.

Although doctors themselves may feel that they are not sufficiently appreciated by patients, the evidence from the other side, obtained by actually asking people how they regard their doctors, does not support these anxieties. Most patients have a high opinion of their own GP, considering him to be skilful, hardworking, devoted and with a genuine personal interest in them. If he is late for appointments or examines them somewhat hurriedly they will generously attribute any such defects to the pressing nature of his commitments in the continual battle against diseases more dramatic than their own. One index of patients' satisfaction is the comparative rarity with which people change their practitioner, although they are entitled to do so and the actual procedure is relatively simple. At least, in the eyes of most patients, the doctor's status is still assured.

But even within one occupational group, in this case

medicine, there are different levels of prestige, and a further element in doctors' recent dissatisfactions relates to the relatively lowly position which general practice has held as compared with hospital medicine. The latter is seen as possessing the maximum intellectual excitement and glamour, and the specialist, whether he is a surgeon, physician or obstetrician, can aspire both to more public prestige and acclaim and more in the way of tangible rewards. Some doctors in practice have resented the necessity for passing on most of their interesting cases to specialists who, in accepting these patients for investigation and treatment, are sometimes rather condescending about the general practitioner's previous efforts at diagnosis. The family doctor has come to feel that he is forced to operate at a lower level than hospital doctors, cut off from the mainstream of medical research and prevented by circumstances from fully developing his own potential. Even within the hospital, inter-tribal medical conflicts are discernible, notably between the junior hospital doctors and senior consultants.

Future of general practice

These various professional grievances, which have some basis in fact, have partly contributed to the reorganisation of the health services, which administratively draws together the separate branches which have hitherto been covered by general practice, the hospitals and the local authority health departments. The future pattern of general practice in Britain will involve several doctors working together, in a health centre or polyclinic which is also staffed by nurses, midwives, health visitors, social workers, secretarial staff and other personnel. This new development will improve doctors' working conditions in many respects but it will also raise fresh problems for all concerned and will be likely to alter the general practitioner's image in the eyes of the community.

In future it will be exceptional for a doctor to work alone, building up a one-to-one relationship with each of his patients. The new organisation will deploy different types of staff for special purposes, each using their own skills in the interest of patients and their families. These health centres will be much more complex than the old type of general practice and will face some of the organisational difficulties of large-scale health care institutions, like hospitals.

Health centres

In the first place, within the new centres, there is bound to be the question as to who is to be the overall administrator. Not all doctors have either the desire or the ability to act in this capacity. The organisation of a health centre serving a population of up to thirty or forty thousand people is a major undertaking. Yet where a lay administrator is appointed his decision may not command the respect of the doctors who, because of their sense of superior professional status, may limit or call in question some of his policy decisions. But trained administrators who are also doctors may not be available in sufficient numbers.

Then, within the organisation itself, hierarchies are bound to develop. Even the group of doctors may experience intra-professional jealousies if it is felt that some among them are gaining special privileges in respect of powers to make decisions, the use of staff, extra space or leisure opportunities. It may prove best, in practice, to have several smaller groups of doctors. Depending on the categories of community nurses and other staff who are working under the same roof, parallel lines of authority will also exist within the centre and the doctors will not be able to assume that others who are employed there will automatically obey their orders and accept their lead. The administration of the nursing side is under close consideration and, in some cases, the senior management involved may also have responsibility for some hospital staff.

Secondly, as far as the doctors' relationships with patients are concerned, it will no longer be the case that a patient can always see the same member of the team. The doctors' timetables will have to be carefully planned and patients who turn up for attention will have to be dealt with by whoever is on duty at the time. A very important point, for the patient, will be whether such centres supply a round-the-clock service.

This reorganisation of the medical services in Britain has ostensibly been undertaken in order to deliver the highest quality of skilled medical care in the most efficient and economic manner to all patients in the community. So health centres have been planned as large units, which will justify the allocation to them of nursing and social work staffs, and the heavy expenditure which special laboratory and diagnostic facilities entail. As well as dealing with the current medical needs of patients and their families, the new centres will also be actively concerned with preventive medicine, endeavouring by education, immunisation and early attention to warning signs of ill health, to raise the general standard of health of the community. The facilities which are offered, in terms of equipment and specialised assistance, will be far more lavish than doctors in practice have previously known. However, in the process, the image of the doctor held by society is bound to change, so that he becomes less of a powerful father figure to whom one's personal woes and sins are confessed and more of a highly skilled, scientific diagnostician controlling a team of experts dealing with a set of medical and social problems.

Change in doctor's image

Another potent influence contributing to a change in the public image of the doctor is television, where the

93

doctor is habitually featured against a formidable array of instruments in a laboratory or the paraphernalia of an operating theatre. At the same time the media produces some programmes which show the doctor as the embodiment of common social values, giving sound practical advice on how to cope with various crises and life experiences. This is in contrast to the old picture of the physician as a charismatic personality with superhuman, priestly powers, challenging death and disaster. He has been, as it were, cut down to size and now accords more appropriately with the secular age in which he functions.

There are other factors which contribute to the demystification of medicine. Most modern treatment is so successful that, in many cases, patients scarcely realise the peril they have encountered and underestimate the skills which went to make their recovery possible. For example, many diseases, once rightly dreaded, are now either prevented or so rapidly treated that their threat is virtually forgotten. Examples are lobar pneumonia, meningitis, blood poisoning, pernicious anaemia, tuberculosis, congenital syphilis and many infectious diseases of childhood. The manifestations of many illnesses can now only be learnt by medical students from textbooks, since florid 'cases' are never permitted to run their natural course. If doctors themselves can scarcely comprehend what certain illnesses were like in the days before modern drugs it is scarcely surprising that patients should be unaware of a passing brush with death.

It is much rarer for families nowadays to experience the disruption and distress which a long illness, nursed at home, used to involve. In fact, the old style doctor could do little more than try all kinds of supportive treatments, in the form of emetics and tonics, poultices, infusions and inhalations and mild or stimulating diets. Yet his constant presence in such a case was an infinite source of reassurance both to the distressed relatives and to the weakened patient and his authority was undoubtedly reinforced in the process. It should not be forgotten, however, that only a small proportion of well-to-do families could afford the ministrations of a personal physician.

A great deal of sickness today is much less dramatic than formerly, partly because of the success of scientific medicine in certain fields and partly because we know more about prevention, but also because our population now lives to encounter the so-called 'degenerative diseases', which affect a middle-aged and elderly population. Many such illnesses are gradually progressive in their effects. Chronic bronchitis, rheumatism and mental illness, for example, all manifest themselves recurrently, they may get a little worse or a little better, but medical treatment, though undoubtedly of help, can seldom effect a lasting cure. There are still potentially fatal conditions in which the doctor's prompt, early action and continuing attention are of the utmost importance, notably in the case of heart attacks and cancer. But many of the symptoms which patients bring to their doctors are more disabling than deadly and simply require to be relieved by a range of easily available medicaments, at little cost to the patient except in terms of time.

As a result of all these developments, the doctor in ordinary general practice has inevitably lost some of the aura which surrounds those who daily fight with death. The acutely ill are generally removed to hospital whilst those who die at home are often so old that their relatives have come to terms with the basic unlikelihood of cure. In other words, the ordinary doctor has now to depend more and more for his authority upon his scientific knowledge, whilst the additional attribute of charisma attaches preeminently to the specialist and, above all, to the surgeon.

Community medicine specialist

Before leaving the theme of the doctor in society, a word is appropriate about a new kind of physician, the community medical specialist. The great majority of doctors are involved with individual patients, applying their skills and experience to diagnose clinical problems and making decisions which affect particular people's lives. But certain doctors are trained to consider the medical needs of communities, in statistical terms. Their speciality is sometimes called population medicine or social medicine and it is concerned with the condition of large groups of people, taking into account all the factors in their physical and social environment which have led to their developing certain illnesses or disabilities. The community medicine specialist will concentrate on preventive medicine; he will also be a kind of medical accountant, making up balance sheets in which the numbers of people in any community with various illnesses are compared with the available resources, in terms of the total numbers of doctors, nurses, hospital beds and so on. Doctors like these have a very important part to play in the health service but, because of their comparative remoteness and the impersonal nature of their tasks, they can expect little in the way of public acclaim.

The sick person seeks a satisfying explanation of his own personal illness or misfortune and is supremely indifferent to the kind of information which statistics supplies. When someone is incapacitated he wants specific advice, a precise prescription, a set of orders which, if they are conscientiously followed, will ensure recovery. They want to 'hand over' to a doctor who will understand their case and deal with it in his wisdom, if necessary, issuing them with orders which they must meticulously obey. It is very much easier for a clinical doctor to persuade patients to take their treatment during an illness than for a doctor who is an enthusiast for preventive medicine to persuade people in the community to abandon habits which are injurious to health.

One of the doctor's very newest tasks is the discovery of premonitory signs of illness among groups of people who are specially at risk to certain diseases. This is a difficult and complicated concept. It is not easy for doctors to take on such a role and it also requires a changed attitude on the part of the community. But our affluent and well-doctored society is already abandoning the fears appropriate to an age in which sudden death and severe illness were commonplace at all ages, and we are beginning to expect skilled help for all kinds of ailments which might never previously have reached professional notice.

People will always need doctors, illnesses will never be completely eradicated and death comes to everyone. Because of this, the doctor's basic position in society is secure. But even the ancient medical profession is not immune to change and doctors must be prepared to adapt to new circumstances, to welcome new colleagues and to co-operate in new arrangements for the provision of medical care.

Questions

1 What were the original three branches of medicine in Britain?
2 What are the main points on which medical ethics rests?
3 There are certain situations in which a doctor's duty to his patient may be unclear. Describe some of these.
4 Mention some different kinds of doctors and say which of them you consider most impress the general public.
5 Most doctors have to undergo a long and expensive training. Do you consider that this is always necessary, for example, in developing countries with large populations and limited resources?
6 Give some reasons why doctors are usually respected by the society in which they practise.
7 What are the dangers of granting a lot of authority to one profession?
8 Contrast the ways of working of a GP working single-handed and a doctor in a large health centre. Which of these do you suppose make most use of nurses' skills?

9 In what ways are the attitudes of the public towards doctors changing? What factors have contributed to these changes?

Further reading

BLOOM, SAMUEL W. (1966) 'The process of becoming a physician', in *A Sociological Framework for Patient Care*, eds J. R. Folta and E. Deck, John Wiley, New York.

CARTWRIGHT, ANN (1967) *Patients and their Doctors: A Study of General Practice*, Reports of the Institute of Community Studies, Routledge & Kegan Paul, London.

JACO, E. G. (1958) ed., *Patients, Physicians and Illness*, Free Press, Chicago.

OSMOND, HUMPHREY (1966) 'Honor a physician? Some thoughts upon the doctor-patient relationship', *Journal of the Medical Society of New Jersey, 63*, 512-18.

SIGERIST, HENRY E. (1960) 'The physician and his environment', from *On the Sociology of Medicine*, ed. M. I. Roemer, M.D. Publications, New York.

SUSSER, M. W. and WATSON, W. (1971) *Sociology in Medicine*, Ch. 7, 'Medicine and bureaucracy', Oxford University Press, London.

The New General Practice II (1970), articles published in the *British Medical Journal*.

Primary Medical Care (1970) Planning Unit Report No 4, British Medical Association, BMA House, London.

V The hospital

Three streams of authority within hospitals; nursing management, bureaucratic structure, clearly defined roles and status levels; organisation of medical staff, supposed equality, actual differences in power of certain doctors; the lay administration; ways of improving co-operation between separate authorities; patients in hospital, their fundamental fears and discontents; development of concern with better communications; patients' demand for and right to information; childbirth in our culture, risk of depersonalisation in obstetric practice; morale and effectiveness in general hospitals; the special care of the dying; the young child in hospital; the mentally handicapped in institutions, arguments regarding most appropriate care; general conclusions regarding provisions for long-term disability.

Streams of authority

The modern hospital is an extremely complex organisation, often employing hundreds of people with widely different skills and functions, who all make some contribution, however small and indirect towards patient care. Most of this chapter will concentrate upon the situation of different sick people in institutions, but first we must take a look at the administration of medical and nursing care because this will help to put the nurse's position into perspective and relate it both to the patients whom she serves and to the medical staff with whom she works. The nurse, as we have seen, has primarily a caring function and it is she who must co-ordinate many of the elements of treatment in the interests of the comfort and well-being of her patients.

The most difficult and fundamental questions regarding hospitals have to do with the quality of the care which patients receive and this matter is certainly not limited to medical treatment but is dependent upon the interactions and co-operation of all who are involved in the management of the sick. The hospital can be viewed as a social environment within which many groups of people are at work and, in order for nurses to operate effectively for the benefit of patients, they need to be aware of how various different occupational groups regard their own functions and how they go about achieving their separate aims. Space will not allow us to consider all who are employed in hospitals, but it is clear that nursing management, the medical power structure and the lay administration are all of central importance. So these will be discussed before going on to consider certain categories of patients whose needs deserve separate attention.

As previous chapters have indicated, the process of becoming a nurse or midwife or doctor produces individuals with clear social responsibilities whose common experience has fostered feelings of loyalty between colleagues who have experienced the same training and now hold similar ideals. While the aspiring nurse, midwife or medical undergraduate is in training, they accept the guidance of their teachers in both theoretical and practical matters, respecting the wisdom of qualified seniors who are possessed of superior knowledge on all aspects of their chosen field of work. But the nurse or midwife, even while technically a student, has also to accept authority of a kind which her opposite number, the medical student, scarcely encounters. The student or pupil nurse or midwife is obliged to carry out orders issued by her superiors, who delegate to her certain tasks for which she is personally responsible. This authority is built into the structure of the nursing profession at all levels, affecting those in training as well as those who are fully qualified. It is not merely a matter of the trainee nurse or midwife being advised to make a bed in a particular way or listening to a description of the correct manner of taking a pulse. Once on the wards she is under an obligation to carry out a number of tasks which a superior officer issues and she must obey these commands to the best of her ability. The nurse or midwife in training can seldom dissociate her student role from her role as an essential member of the ward staff who will be called upon to execute tasks according to precise instructions. The kind of jobs she is asked to do should, of course, be suited to her level of knowledge and her experience, but they all form a part of the actual care of patients. Nurses learn on the job and their labour contributes sizably to the total man or womanpower available in any hospital which undertakes training courses.

Nursing management

In the discussion in Chapter III of the revolution which came about in nursing practice one hundred years ago, it was pointed out how the increasing specialisation and precision of medicine came to require a corresponding sophistication in nursing techniques, rendering inadequate the former simple ministrations of relatives and untrained ward hands, and making it essential that the prescribed treatment of patients should continue smoothly in the physician's absence. The need for more efficient patient care prompted both nurse training and the hierarchy which divided and distributed the responsibility for the provision of care. The multiplication of nursing grades has continued ever since and, even during her studentship, the hospital nurse is bound to experience something of the military style discipline to which she will always thereafter be subject. It is quite exceptional, even in the field of private nursing, for any individual to avoid the ranking of nursing grades which is characteristic of the profession.

Bureaucratic structure

The necessity for what is essentially a bureaucratic organisation of different ranks of staff comes about, not only on account of the magnitude and complexity of nursing tasks, but because there are so many nurses in any hospital that some division of responsibilities is inevitable. As soon as the stage was past when one old-time physician could descend upon a ward and issue a few practical admonitions to one solitary maid of all work, as soon as there was even one more so-called 'nurse' on the premises, some delegation of duties had to take place. As staff increased to match the work load, the ward sister became the person 'in charge' of the total nursing operations and proceeded to the rational allocation of available personnel among the assembled patients and their needs.

Until recently, the pattern of nursing organisation most commonly encountered had, at the top, the matron with her assistant and deputies beneath her. These high ranking individuals did no practical nursing but saw to it that staff and resources were available to ensure the care of all the patients. The matron's regular rounds of the entire hospital drew attention to her symbolic headship of the nurses and her overall concern for the patients. Then, below the nursing administrators, were a number of ward sisters, all of equivalent status and each responsible for nursing matters within her own ward. The sisters supervised the great bulk of the practical staff, who could be of several types, including, possibly, staff nurses who were already registered nurses, nurses in training, enrolled nurses, pupil nurses as well as various grades of untrained or auxiliary staff.

Clearly defined roles

It is a notable characteristic of hospital society that, with the exception of the sister and the staff nurse, the majority of the nurses on the wards are usually in a state of change. For example, those in training are liable to move away in the course of gaining experience in a variety of clinical settings; then there are constant changes in personnel because of the shift system, to allow for time off duty; in addition, some nurses will leave, on the completion of training or for personal reasons, and be replaced by others. One of the objects of strict hierarchy, with the duties at each level well defined, is to get over the ever present problem of changing staff. Thus, if one particular individual moves they are promptly replaced by another who carries on with exactly the same job. The capacity to perform particular tasks and take on definite responsibilities resides not in the individual nurse but in her achieved role. The attribute must belong to the status which the worker has achieved so that, when one person drops out, another can carry on the tasks, exactly as though no change had occurred.

It is clear that the organisation of this aspect of the nursing service alone, namely the provision of an effective corps on duty throughout every twenty-four hours, requires very careful planning and the operation of special skills. Add to this the supply and distribution of material as well as human resources, medicines, appliances, equipment, clothing and so on, and the task of nursing management becomes still more complex. Meanwhile, a never ending stream of patients, each with unique requirements in respect of medication, special nursing care and monitoring, must have all their needs co-ordinated and fulfilled in accord with tight schedules whose precision is an integral part of the treatment. The responsible nurse has often to work under considerable pressure, making rapid decisions over a wide field and being subject at the same time to innumerable interruptions and unexpected demands from many people.

Recently, the administration of nursing has been modified, allowing nurses with more experience to be given wider responsibilities than one ward can provide. Since the publication of the Salmon Report, a series of numbered ranks have been introduced in higher nursing management. Responsibility at senior levels is now apportioned so that certain senior nursing officers are responsible, in middle management, for groups of wards; still higher are principal nursing officers, equivalent to former matrons, in charge of hospitals, whilst chief nursing officers administer entire groups of hospitals. The officer grades from six to ten each have their jobs specified quite precisely, so that everyone knows their place in the total system and how they relate to those nurses above or below them on the scale. Thus, apart from the highest ranking officers, each grade has a nurse above her who can, within limits, tell her what to do whilst she herself can issue instructions to and supervise a number of nurses who are immediately inferior to her. The system has necessitated special training courses in nursing management to accustom the participants to its operation and demonstrate its advantages to the profession.

The recent concentration upon the re-organisation of senior nursing structure has possibly tended to convey the impression to outsiders that the status system is becoming an end in itself instead of being a means to better patient care. In this respect, nursing administration runs the risks of any bureaucracy, where the rule book may become supreme. The profession, as a whole, has welcomed the change. It is too soon to judge how effectively a tightly knit officer corps can overcome the continuing problems which many hospitals experience of being partly dependent upon heterogeneous 'other nursing staff'. Efficiency in senior administration will not automatically bring about improved standards in patient care at the bedside. The latter is notoriously difficult to measure, but deserves more attention than it has hitherto received, even if this means taking into account the medical as well as the nursing components. It is clearly easier for a profession to review its internal relationships, introducing incentives and improving career prospects, than to face the confusions of its infra-structure or the resistance of a rival professional group. However, the Briggs Report has lately definitely contributed to new thinking in this field and has placed the emphasis firmly upon patient needs.

Limitations of authoritarian pattern

Another pertinent consideration is to ask how far a very
authoritarian pattern is appropriate to all classes of patient.
The new administrative structure applies across the board,
out in the community and in institutions caring for the
chronically sick and disabled, as well as to intensive cardiac
care units, neo-natal units and hospitals for the acutely
ill. In places where precision is essential and time is at a
premium, a military style operation has obvious advantages.
There is simply no room for individual variation and possible error and the medical and senior nursing personnel
rightly expect prompt, standardised responses to demands.
But this is far from the situation in which many of today's
hospitalised patients exist and there should be opportunities
for more experiments in both staffing and physical structure. The recent administrative changes are, in effect, a
further elaboration of the former regime, which was based
firmly upon physical ward units, within which all the
patients' activities were confined.

Recently there has been a lot of somewhat vague talk
of the 'team' approach to nursing in hospitals. This seems
to mean an arrangement whereby specified groups of nurses
from the available ward staff will concentrate upon the care
of a limited number of patients, and the implication is that
this will promote better care for the patients as well as
more satisfaction for the nurses concerned. It is, however,
very difficult to envisage how such teams would differ in
practice from the existing ward structure. Each small team
within a ward would need a leader of maximum seniority
and experience who would deploy the activities of a series
of subordinate nurses and aides, according to their proven
abilities. This looks like the logical downwards extension
of the principle of delegation of responsibility. But such a
redefinition of internal relationships need not, in itself, alter
nurses' relationships with patients.

It is somewhat paradoxical that a highly formalised status

system should have to be elaborated to deal with the vagaries of human illness, disablement and misfortune. The structure is supposedly devised in response to the problems of those sick people who cannot be adequately cared for by their families. A high proportion of in-patients today are elderly and most hospital beds in this country are occupied by the mentally ill or disabled. Yet society and the nursing and medical professions often continue to think in late-nineteenth-century terms with a limited conception of the hospital's functions. There should, in future, be a wider graduation of curing and caring institutions, with a range of environments suited to the needs of those members of society who are temporarily or permanently unable to manage at home. It is debatable whether nurses need staff all such places or whether the capacity and readiness to care is the nurse's exclusive preserve. We shall return to this problem later, in relation to certain of the disabled.

Organisation of medical staff

Turning now from nurses to doctors, the hospital provides them with a prominent stage upon which they can perform their dramatic roles before mixed audiences, who observe all their activities with intense interest. Although, as will be seen, doctors ostensibly decry authority within their own profession, they are the group who effectively possess the maximum power within hospitals, superseding their highly organised nursing colleagues and leaving the lay administration far behind.

The reason for this state of affairs is not difficult to comprehend, since it is the doctors who, in the course of diagnosing illness and prescribing treatment make the key decisions in hospital and issue the central commands. In coming to a diagnosis the doctor will naturally be aided by information provided by the nursing staff as well as by the results of various special investigations, but the analysis of this data and the conclusions to be drawn from it

106

ultimately depend upon the doctor himself. Similarly, the subsequent stage of laying down a therapeutic regime is his prerogative, even although the actual organisation and administration of treatment as well as the observation and recording of the patient's responses will largely fall to nurses. In other words, the physician initiates the key activities which take place in hospitals and contacts those members of the nursing staff who are sufficiently competent and senior to ensure (by appropriate delegation) that treatment is carried out. This does not detract from the very great importance of skilled nursing care and its effect upon patients, both in wards for the acutely ill and in institutions for the chronically sick. Nevertheless, the fact remains that, though the doctor's visits may be brief and infrequent, he is the primary agent of change, initiating, altering or stopping treatment, deciding to admit this person and to discharge the next, thereby affecting both his patients' lives and the nature of the nurse's tasks.

Supposed equality of doctors

As the last chapter suggested, the sole justification for the very lengthy and intensive training which a doctor undergoes, with its accompanying tests and examinations, is to produce someone who will be skilled in diagnosis, prognosis, prevention and treatment of illness. This is what society demands of him and, once he has been registered, they accept him as being competent to practise. Provided that he does not transgress the profession's ethical code, no other doctor can order him how to carry out his job. Theoretically, all registered medical practitioners are of equal rank. The addition of a specialist qualification supposedly makes no difference to the nature of this relationship between doctors. Obviously, however, it does greatly alter the range of their work in practice, the size of their financial rewards and the respect which they are accorded by patients and fellow practitioners.

In the hospital setting, when a consultant is apparently 'telling' the resident doctor or registrar how to treat a patient, a different kind of process is taking place from that in which the sister tells the student nurse her duties. The kind of authority which the consultant is using derives from his superior knowledge or experience and is essentially in the nature of advice, not an order. The very word 'consultant' indicates that he is a person whom other doctors consult in search of helpful advice. He has access to special knowledge useful to the care of the patient, but the younger doctor is under no formal obligation to take the advice, which can theoretically be disputed or rejected. Of course, in the great majority of cases, the consultant's word is, in fact, taken as law, but this does not alter the nature of the communication between colleagues. Moreover, once the consultant departs, the doctor on the ward is expected to employ his own discretion and initiative in the management of patients and must make the necessary decisions in the event of any emergency. Although junior doctors usually do defer to their seniors, upon whom they depend ultimately for references and preferment, and although they often resent their conditions of work, there is no comparable bureaucratic organisation on the medical side of a hospital to that which exists on the nursing side. The medical hierarchy ultimately depends upon tacit agreement rather than on a system of ranks and job specifications.

Actual prestige levels

At the same time, it must be granted that some medical roles are more glamorous and desirable than others. The surgeon performs in a theatre which is fraught with drama for all the participants and which the general public love to contemplate, at a safe distance, through the media. Medical students frequently hope to become surgeons and, contrariwise, they often despise psychiatry and social medicine. Within the ranks of surgeons, a particularly telling

tour de force by one specialist may set off a chain reaction
of transplant operations throughout the world, all calculated to ensure the maximum publicity, if not the optimum therapeutic results. Doctors who dice with the death
of their patients occupy a special social pedestal and enjoy
rewards of fame to which the faithful physicians of the
chronically sick can seldom aspire. The behaviour of surgeons in the midst of their chosen scene of action has been
graphically portrayed by Goffman. He points out that during an operation the central actor in the drama is, to all
intents and purposes, absent, being under an anaesthetic,
and so doctors are free to talk about him in a manner which
would be considered quite improper at the bedside. It is
interesting to extend this observation to the situation of
patients who, from the point of view of the medical staff,
are sometimes spoken of as though they were not present,
such as the terminally ill, the psychotic, the mentally subnormal and those patients who are wheeled, apparently
comatose, into accident and emergency departments. But,
since this section of the chapter is mainly concerned with
staff rather than patients, we will now turn to the third
main element in hospital organisation, the lay administration.

Lay administration

The third element in the organisation of hospitals in Britain
is the lay administration, headed by a medical superintendent who is an employee of the relevant health board,
hospital board or committee of management. He is broadly
responsible for the financial affairs of the hospital and,
through his staff, administers the material side of an institution which requires in many respects, to be managed
like a large hotel. The medical superintendent presides
over subordinate staff who are bound to follow his instructions and who have clearly defined duties. In effect, he
heads a bureaucratic organisation which is more similar

in structure to the nursing hierarchy than it is to the group-
ing of independent doctors who constitute the medical
staff.

Because the medical staff have been brought up to the
expectation of power and the exercise of responsibility,
they tend to favour the dictates of their own professional
consciences and they do not prove easily amenable to
direction by the lay administration. Thus, although the
medical superintendent may be the titular head of the
institution, conveying the wishes and will of management
committee or more distant board, his powers of command
are, in fact, strictly limited, positioned as he is between
the highly-organised nursing staff on the one hand and a
set of idiosyncratic consultants on the other. Even if the
superintendent is a doctor himself his position is not rendered much easier since, as we have seen, this gives him
no automatic power to command his colleagues, who continue to preside over their several empires and who will
always tend to regard a clinical specialist qualification as
being superior to the command of administrative skills.

Communication difficulties

Various devices are employed in order to reduce some
of the difficulties in communication between these three
parallel lines of command in hospitals, such as regular
meetings at which all are represented. However, it frequently happens, even at this policy level, that the consultants contrive to have their own way whilst, at ward
level, the individual doctor continues to make direct contact with the ward sister or equivalent nursing officer regarding the detailed treatment of the patients for whom he
is responsible.

Professional co-operation

In practice there are many situations where nurses and

110

doctors co-operate closely and where questions of professional precedence are irrelevant. For example, the sister in charge of a special unit for premature babies will be accepted as an expert by the doctors with whom she works and much of the success of treatment will depend upon her skill and vigilance. As we have seen, this skill is not merely a matter of personal competence but the ability to deploy all her staff to the optimum advantage. When the pace in a ward is fairly leisurely and questions relate to long-term care rather than to sudden, medical intervention, nurses are likely to have a major say in the decisions which are made. The contrasting situation is an emergency when medical and nursing staff will be galvanised into co-operative action on the patient's behalf and professional disagreements will be forgotten in the common effort to save life or limbs. Midwives are empowered to conduct deliveries and will rightly do so in the absence of an obstetrician. Clearly, the availability of different grades of nursing or auxiliary staff will determine the actual distribution of the work which must be done and nurses will not stand upon ceremony or claim exemption by reason of status when their patients are in need.

However these matters of relationship and duties are resolved in any particular instance, doctors and nurses share a familiar working environment. Rosen has called the hospital a 'health workshop'. It is a place in which the staff play accepted roles and within which they hope to achieve long-term and short-term professional goals. They may not be conscious of the intricacies of its administration or realise how many separate groups interact and compete within its walls. But their own membership of the hospital staff places them in a position of relative influence and gives all of them some chance to make decisions affecting their own personal prospects and the welfare of those in their care.

The patient in hospital

However, the patient who has to enter hospital is in a very different situation and he is liable to view his setting in a totally different light. For him the occasion is surrounded with uncertainty and fear. Worries connected with his immediate illness are compounded by ignorance regarding its possible outcome and duration and the effect upon others of his incapacity. Meanwhile, his strange new surroundings, peopled by a confusing multitude of actors whose roles he can scarcely imagine, add to his general uneasiness and sense of helplessness.

It is easy for both doctors and nurses to be preoccupied with accomplishing their immediate tasks and with conveying an impression of competence or infallibility to their colleagues, patients and superiors and, indeed, the life of a hospital offers many rewards in terms of job satisfaction and social encounters. But the student nurse can also be rendered very anxious by the sort of work she has to do, the situations she encounters and her limited understanding of the reasons for her activities. It is useful to reiterate what is her primary function, as the person who supplies patients in hospital with all the basic elements necessary to support life. She must ensure that they are kept safe, warm, fed, clean and rested, thus providing the conditions most conducive to their cure and comfort, and she must co-ordinate all the separate elements in their treatment.

The patient's optimum comfort involves peace of mind and this is something which the nurse, more than anyone else, should be in a position to ensure. The doctor's contact with the patient may be highly significant, determining stages in the hospital cycle from admission through diagnosis and treatment to discharge but, because he has to distribute his skills among so many individuals, the time which he can spend with any one person is necessarily brief. Nurses, who theoretically, come into much more prolonged contact with each patient, should be able to uncover and, if possible, allay their worries as well as tending to their bodily needs. If nurses are to become patient-orientated rather than concentrating upon specific tasks, they need to have some insight into what a period in hospital can mean to different people. There is already a considerable amount of information available on this important subject drawn from numerous studies among patients in a variety of settings. In addition, however, nurses must appreciate some of the reasons for their own personal reluctance to contemplate disturbing human emotions and be aware of the practical limitations which ward routine can put upon relations with patients.

The sociological approach to studying patients in hospital involves a search for common patterns of behaviour characteristic of certain groups of people. By breaking down the subject in this way more can be learnt than by simply taking each case separately. It is, for instance, a considerable oversimplification to refer to 'the patient in hospital' since both patients and hospitals vary enormously. Those in surgical units experience personal crises of a different nature and intensity from patients in the less dramatic setting of the medical wards. Hospitals for the acutely ill provide environments which contrast markedly with institutions designed for the care or containment of the chronically sick and the mentally disturbed. Women who go into hospitals for delivery are in an entirely different category from women who enter hospital to die. The very old and the very young both dislike strange people and surroundings, so small children and old people may be seriously disturbed by a hospital admission. The atmosphere in an isolation hospital, as its name implies, is likely to add loneliness to antisepsis, whereas a day hospital can be virtually a home from home.

It was not until the 1960s that interest was aroused in this country regarding the question of patients' reactions to treatment. Remember that the majority of effective drugs and antibiotics only became generally available after the

113

Second World War. Then, after the introduction of the National Health Service in 1948, there was an accumulation of unmet physical needs to be met in the patient population and doctors were understandably engrossed in the business of coping with symptoms and syndromes which had previously been unmanageable. By the time the health service had been in operation for a dozen years, doctors and administrators were still reluctant to admit that the mere provision of a free service would not automatically provide complete satisfaction for all insured consumers. Formerly, poor patients had been fortunate to secure admission to institutions maintained by philanthropists or parish relief, but treatment was now open to every citizen as a right and hospital patients ought no longer to be regarded as objects of charity. Gradually the medical profession realised that some patients were not fully content with the circumstances of their hospital care and that they had quite specific complaints and criticisms to put forward.

Communications in hospital

At this time the word 'communication' was much in vogue, and a medical and nursing advisory committee produced a report on 'Communication between doctors, nurses and patients' in which they spotlighted this neglected aspect of human relations within hospitals. They mildly suggested that nearly all patients wanted and were entitled to know more about their medical condition and that positive steps should be taken to supply them with information on their diagnosis, prognosis, and treatment.

It had always been the case, of course, that the wealthy, whether treated at home or in a nursing home, were at liberty to discuss their condition at length with their own personal physician or chosen specialist. But there had been a tendency to take a somewhat different line with the

114

poorer and less educated unfortunates who were admitted to charity institutions. The former habits of patronising condescension were seen to be singularly inappropriate and offensive within the new health service. The ordinary patient's right to treatment should, it was now maintained, be paralleled by a right to knowledge, especially about matters vital to their own and their families' well-being.

This latter consideration, namely the fact that patients did not exist in a social vacuum but had families in the world outside, had also been slow in penetrating official and professional consciousness, but at last the influence which social factors could have upon the manifestation and nature of much current illness was being increasingly recognised. The naïve hopes that the health service would serve to diminish the demand for medical care had been proved totally unfounded, and this forced official consideration of the social setting of symptomatology.

In addition, there was growing awareness of the unfortunate divisions between separate sections of the existing health service and, in particular, of the way in which the hospital's activities and its staff were virtually insulated from the surrounding community. A patient could at times leave hospital, not only lacking personal knowledge of his own condition, but without his general practitioner being notified or adequately informed. A nursing study by Muriel Skeet, entitled *Home from Hospital,* bore awful witness to the real neglect which could occur because of administrative gaps in the service.

For all these reasons, an attempt was finally made to analyse the meaning of a hospital admission for the people whom the hospital aimed to serve. But the motives for tackling this neglected area of human relations were not entirely altruistic, since the medical profession had meanwhile become thoroughly alarmed by the pressing nature of some patients' complaints and had decided that an attempt to explain what went on in hospitals was urgently needed from the point of view of better public relations. In

115

other words, improved communications might forestall litigation.

Following the publication of the above-mentioned advisory committee's report, a number of investigations were undertaken to supplement the little that was then known or conjectured about patients' views of the hospital service. The largest of these, by Ann Cartwright, involved interviewing a random sample of over seven hundred people, from all over England and Wales, who had once been in hospital, whether as surgical patients, medical patients or for confinement. At the same time, a noteworthy study into the morale and effectiveness of general hospitals was carried out by Revans in the Manchester area and, subsequently, some of the recommendations which it offered were tried out in practice elsewhere.

Patients' attitudes

Since then there have been many smaller investigations in all kinds of hospitals so that we are now in a position to draw some general conclusions. Whereas some studies have been purely descriptive, others have tried to assess the therapeutic effect of a deliberate policy to modify the behaviour of hospital staff towards patients. So the subject has now progressed beyond the stage of academic interest and has resulted, in some quarters, in positive efforts to alter the patients' environment by what can appropriately be termed 'therapeutic behaviour'. First, however, let us review what has been discovered about the attitudes of patients in hospital, leaving till later the consideration of nursing attitudes and the possibility of their modification.

It is now well established that the events leading up to a hospital admission can be accompanied by a great deal of anxiety, frustration and delay. Part of the delay may be the patients' own fault, but some people may have to wait months before finally being given an appointment with a consultant and being allowed to join a long queue in an uncomfortable out-patient department. Eventually the specialist assesses the need for hospital care and admission may be arranged.

Admission procedure

The actual process of entry to hospital can be a disturbing experience. At a time when the patient is uncertain of what to expect, when his relatives have left or are about to depart, he may be faced by someone whose main interest seems to be in coldly recording his identity in terms of name, address and religion. He is quite likely to have to undress to order and get into bed, whilst his day time garments are discreetly removed or concealed. Thus deprived of many of his most personal attributes and supports, he contemplates his strange surroundings.

In an emergency, the time scale is entirely different and the inevitable sense of urgency may serve to heighten the patient's existing pain and distress. The admission procedure, moreover, will probably still seem alarmingly impersonal, an impression accentuated by brusque commands of nurses or doctors to porters. Orders like, 'Wheel over the male collapse' or, 'Bring in the acute female now' are not calculated to improve the patient's morale if he is capable of appreciating what is afoot.

In several respects, admission to an institution involves a loss of identity and a reduction in status. The patient has to relinquish the people and possessions which ordinarily reflect and express his own personality and reinforce his sense of uniqueness and importance. His achieved position in society now counts for nothing since he is there in the ward by virtue of an accidental bodily failing, for which he can claim no credit but which can be of consuming interest to his attendants. Suddenly, by becoming an in-patient, he is reduced to a dependent position where he has to rely upon others to supply many of his simplest needs and where his freedom of action is severely restricted. His help-

117

less posture is, of course, complemented by the nurse's dominant position as benevolent provider allied to the doctor's healing role. The features of dependency and change of status are not confined to sick people in hospital, being characteristic of the sick role itself. However, the hospital emphasises both features, because the ward and its staff are visible evidence of the patient's altered and abnormal role, whereas a familiar home environment can sustain a sense of continuity.

Patients vary in their tolerance of dependency. Some find it reassuring to be completely taken care of and to be temporarily treated like small children affords them an atavistic pleasure, but others fret over their enforced impotence and deeply resent being ordered about and patronised. Whatever their basic reaction to the sick role, the majority of patients, once they have settled down in the ward, warmly appreciate the nurse's ministrations. Sisters especially are set on a pedestal by the public and singled out for praise. They are usually clearly distinguishable from the mixed and changing group of other ward staff, and they appear as figures clothed in authority and epitomising efficiency. But patients also seem to be aware of the subtle effect which the sister can have in promoting or preventing a relaxed ward atmosphere.

In our affluent society it is possible for many people in their daily lives to be largely insulated from unpleasant sights and experiences and to avoid repulsive or uncongenial companions. But a hospital collects all manner of sick and unfortunate individuals, forcing into close proximity people who would never otherwise come into contact. This can be productive of tension and misunderstanding but, on the whole, the sharing of common misfortunes leads to friendliness and increased concern for others. Loneliness and anxiety are lessened by the opportunity to talk and compare notes. However, a proportion of patients are distressed by the contemplation of suffering and, in particular, by the presence of death. Themselves unable to render any help to the desperately ill or dying, they become very critical of staff attitudes and actions, while they simultaneously feel personally threatened by the sight of another's mortality.

Patients' right to information

In any illness, death is the possibility and recovery the hope. Patients are not qualified to grasp the complexities of diagnosis and treatment or the statistical probabilities upon which prognosis depends. But their medical ignorance is matched by an intense interest in their own condition and a desire to know more about it This definitely does not mean that they want, or should receive, accounts of pathology supplemented by surgery or biochemistry, since these very terms belong to a language foreign to laymen. They are all, quite naturally, anxious to know what their illness implies in terms of likely length of stay in hospital, whether and when they can expect to return completely to 'normal' or how far they may have to modify their mode of life. They want and have a right to be told the probable repercussions of their incapacity upon their family and their work prospects. They speculate endlessly as to why this should have happened to them, what could have 'brought it on', and the kind of answers which they give themselves and one another are far removed from the explanations of scientific medicine. For the patient, illness is a strange and unwanted experience which interrupts their plans and the orderly fabric of their existence. It demands an explanation which will allow them to fit it into some kind of meaningful picture and come to terms with its arbitrary and unpleasant nature.

Many hospitals do issue 'information' sheets or booklets, but these mainly relate to the bread and butter or board and lodging side of hospital life. Designed by administrators, they describe timetables and physical facilities but do not presume to trespass upon medical territory. It is in relation to their medical condition that patients feel the lack of communication most acutely and it is significant that as many as three-fifths of those interviewed in the nationwide survey felt that they had not been told enough about their illness, treatment and prognosis. So there is clear evidence of failure on the part of hospital staff to supply one of their patients' primary demands. We shall look more closely at some of the possible reasons for this presently; meanwhile it is important to realise what a source of dissatisfaction and unhappiness this unrelieved anxiety can represent.

Patient dissatisfaction

When patients are divided into those who are middle class and those who are lower class, it seems at first as if those from the lower class are less concerned about the matter of information. In fact, lower class patients are simply less inclined to ask questions, being at a distinct disadvantage when it comes to putting their worries into words and also being more likely to be over-awed by the medical staff. The most dissatisfied patients of all turn out to be those who want to be told a lot but who do not get round to asking questions. Middle class patients may appear more inquisitive because they are more articulate and more likely to expect technical explanations. Their own education and experience brings them closer to the doctor's way of thinking and speaking and they feel able to address the medical staff on equal terms.

On the other hand, it is the case that a fair number of patients prefer not to be told about their illness. This can be confusing for doctors and nurses, for how are they to distinguish between the people who are not asking for information which they would dearly like and those people for whom ignorance is bliss? Clearly, some patients are prepared to take the hospital on trust, relying upon the doctor's command of medical mysteries to restore them fully to health. Patients also quickly sense the impropriety of asking questions in certain circumstances, a discouraging impression being easily conveyed to them by the attitudes of staff and effectively quelling all but the most persistent enquirers.

Elderly patients are, on the whole, less inclined to ask questions than the young. This may be a consequence of their upbringing since, in their youth, medical care was costly and scarce. But old people generally may feel at a peculiar disadvantage in the confusing and busy hospital scene and may elect to bear humbly their passive role and inferior status. The fatalism of the aged is not confined to traditional cultures.

Childbirth and hospital

In the course of this book we have tended to equate the position of nurses and midwives and this can be defended from the sociological point of view since their differences are less than their similarities. However, the patient's situation as far as maternity hospitals is concerned differs in several important respects from that of patients in general hospitals. In a maternity unit, many of the tasks which the staff perform are routine and repetitive, as hundreds of mothers are steadily processed through the institution from ante-natal clinics to labour wards and on to the lying-in wards. In parts of Britain today over 90 per cent of confinements take place in hospitals and only a minor proportion of cases are likely to need specialised care. So midwifery deals, in the main, with normal people and happy outcomes.

There is something inherently anomalous about treating birth, which is a natural process, in hospitals, with all their connotations of illness, emergency and death. The instrumental paraphernalia of obstetric units, the battery of ante-natal tests, the labour ward rituals and the rules regulating the behaviour of puerperal women all tend to convey the impression that having a child is a matter for experts. Indeed, modern women are often in some considerable doubt as to their status during pregnancy because society persists in treating them as sick in some sense.

There are excellent medical reasons for ensuring that most births should take place in hospital, with trained mid-wives to hand and specialist services available. This arrangement has steadily reduced the numbers of infant deaths in Britain and virtually eliminated maternal mortality. But to cut people off from the family group on the occasion of one of the central events in human life does have social and psychological implications.

In the interests of saving life, the Western world has incidentally neglected human relations. We have been developing this theme in relation to medical care in general, but it applies with special force to the experience of birth and death. In most other cultures the arrival or departure of a member of society is the occasion for elaborate rituals of a kind which support the people most concerned. Not only are most of our babies born in hospital but many mothers in our urbanised society are very ignorant regarding all matters to do with sex and pregnancy and they are unused to handling very small infants. Clearly, if people mainly live in relatively isolated, nuclear family units they will have little opportunity to observe and participate in the process of childbirth and childrearing. Their practical experience in these matters is likely to be extremely limited and based upon childhood memories, whilst the almost universal practice of hospital delivery only makes the matter progressively worse.

It is not surprising that many women enter maternity hospital with considerable apprehension, their basic fears of the unknown being only partly allayed, in some instances, by their prior participation in ante-natal 'classes'. This is an area where the specialists have had more or less to take over completely what was once a rich area of folk

122

wisdom. Old wives' tales have had to be consciously replaced by deliberate attempts to educate by midwives,
doctors and the media. The gain in human lives is
indisputable, but society has not yet found an entirely
satisfactory way of replacing the traditional supports
which formerly assisted the mother through her personal
crisis

Mothers having their first babies, being without previous
personal experience, are obviously the main losers under
the new regime and they are the most likely to complain
about lack of information. These mothers are considerably
apprehensive and are liable to great anxiety throughout
labour. If they are left alone the physical pain which they
experience is exacerbated by fear of more to come and
by their utter helplessness. A woman's perception of time
alters during labour, and what can seem like an age to
her is only a brief period for the busy midwife who has
several patients to attend.

Midwives are the main sources of information and sympathy for women in maternity hospitals. This is not merely
because there are more midwives than doctors, it also
reflects the fact that this is still, in an important sense, a
woman's sphere. Moreover, midwives are empowered by
statute to carry out deliveries unaided. But the midwives
can also come in for considerable criticism, both from the
mother's memories of events in the labour ward, and in
relation to their subsequent experiences. In the grip of
powerful physical forces the labouring woman is easily
oppressed and she may resent what seem to her like un-
concern or callous comments from a young pupil midwife.
To some women, temporarily reduced to an extreme
position of dependency, the brusque exhortations of the
labour ward sister may sound harsh, although others
may welcome the midwife's firm control of the dramatic
situation.

Once her personal ordeal is over, a woman's focus of
attention suddenly changes and starts to centre upon her

helpless infant. She becomes exceedingly sensitive on her baby's behalf, interpreting all kinds of small signs and casual comments as possible portents of disaster. If the baby is kept separate from her or if she is denied the reassurance and physical satisfaction of handling it, her anxiety may increase and be voiced in criticism of the nursing staff. However, it is not enough for the mothers to be left literally 'holding the baby', since many of them need someone to show them in detail how to do it. This is, of course, part of the midwife's role, but if mothers feel they have not had enough help they will again become resentful and dissatisfied.

Because labour and the puerperium are characterised by a heightened sensitivity, with the woman inevitably anxious, first on her own and later on another's account,* the contrast between the personal situation and the impersonal organisation of hospital can be at its most marked. Much can be done to allay the mother's fears, provided that midwives and medical staff are aware of what this outwardly straightforward, routine series of events can mean for the patients concerned. Not only can the nursing staff supply the knowledge and reassurance that the women need but they can encourage the presence of families to provide a warmth which strangers cannot match. It is an interesting comment upon the modern British family that the husband should be the person who is most often offered the dubious privilege of being present at the birth. In other cultures, birth is the occasion for motherly and grandmotherly participation, males being kept some distance from the centre of the drama. Once trained midwives take over from old women, as in our society, the grandmother in the picture is effectively dismissed, and the relevant next of kin becomes the husband. His involvement

* The case of mothers who lose their babies or whose child is born severely deformed or premature requires special attention. Their unhappy situation can be made worse by insensitive placing of them in the midst of normal mothers and babies.

does not always come easily to him and, especially among working class families, grandmothers and female relatives can still be seen to greet new mothers with an effusiveness which the male cannot match.

Morale in hospitals

So far we have been concentrating upon patients' morale in hospitals and how it can be affected by staff attitudes and policies. There is also evidence that nurses are susceptible to atmosphere and that those hospitals where communications between patients and staff are poor also have the highest student nurse wastage. It seems as though in hospitals where consultants are not afraid to discuss their difficulties and uncertainties honestly with the ward sisters, the sisters offer more guidance to their students and these, in turn, talk more openly to the patients. As we have already suggested, it is not only patients who are anxious: hospital nurses and doctors, for all their outward appearance of calm competence, can also be subject to uncertainty.

Revans has proposed that the general anxiety which is a feature of hospital life at all levels can be met in two ways, it can either be denied or admitted. Those in authority may be prepared to admit that they do not know all the answers to all questions, or they may cover up and protect themselves by discouraging awkward questions altogether. Where there is open discussion at higher levels this has the effect of promoting a relaxed atmosphere for junior staff too. This more democratic approach to treatment and teaching ultimately allows the patients more information and more help with expressing their personal anxieties.

In Revan's survey a further most interesting observation emerged: patients in hospitals which had what he termed an open communication climate were being discharged sooner than those who had experienced a unit where discussion was rare. So better communication is not merely an optional extra to medical and nursing care but can be an important part of the total therapy. This point is worth making, as the advocates of improved relations in medical situations are open to the charge of sentimentality and may be accused of promoting irrelevant adjuncts to scientific treatment.

However, to recognise the significance of this element in therapy does not mean that it is easy to introduce. One idea which has been advanced is that each patient should have someone designated as his 'personal doctor' responsible for the personal relations side of the hospital's ministrations and ready to supply all the answers to questions in a suitable form. Others have seen this matter as primarily the nursing sister's responsibility. One deliberate experiment to investigate the effects of specific actions taken to improve communications between patients and hospital staff was notable in its failure to demonstrate any difference at the end of the exercise. Patients were still expressing as much dissatisfaction as before.

But this should come as no surprise, for it is well known that it is difficult to change people's working methods, especially if the old patterns have certain advantages to those concerned. It turns out that, even if ward timetables are altered to allow for more personal contact with patients, nurses may not always take advantage of it. In fact, nurses and doctors are often very reluctant to talk about the patient's most urgent preoccupations and to discuss with him the possible threat to his life which his illness represents. Their brusque and cheerful manner and their tendency to hurry on to the next job can make the patient feel acutely lonely and rejected. It has even been suggested that nurses deliberately arrange ward routines so that, by concentrating on a series of practical tasks which must be performed in a regular, orderly fashion, they may partly avoid the disturbance which individual suffering can occasion. To break up the treatment of any one patient between many different nurses and attendants, all of whom have only a transient contact with him, could be a means of protecting staff from the anxiety which serious illness and death provoke. But it is probably unfair to regard the common pattern of ward organisation as a conspiracy against the person and more sensible to see such routines as a logical development of the original impetus towards orderly management which we have already considered.

Depersonalisation

The more emotional and open approach to patients involves personal relationships with which the young nurse in training may be unwilling and unfitted to deal. She is often expected by her seniors to cultivate a deliberate detachment in the interests of efficiency and is reproved for overt expressions of concern. To an extent, the depersonalisation of nursing and the fact that every job can be done just as well by someone else, is matched by a deliberate depersonalisation of patients. To think of patients as cases of this or that and focusing attention upon their common pathology may mean that their individual hopes and fears are given scant attention. But if any blame is to be fixed for this state of affairs it should fall firmly upon the medical profession which, to date, has been more interested in dealing with physical ills than in altering states of mind. Nurses have always had more inclination towards and training in the general relief of human suffering.

The dying patient

One group of patients in hospital who are likely to experience the greatest failure in communication are those who are perhaps in most need of support, namely the dying. They tend to be unpopular with both doctors and nurses, to whom they are an unwelcome demonstration that medicine can fail and a reminder that all men are mortal. Those who attend the dying often try to make their contacts as brief and superficial as possible and shun encounters which permit the dying person to express his fears. The frequent insistence that such patients should never be told 'the truth' may be a means of protecting the attendant as much as the sick person. It is revealing that a survey among doctors showed that over 80 per cent of them did not believe in telling their dying patients 'the truth', but the same proportion of the doctors would themselves prefer to be told of a fatal prognosis. Our own culture has largely rejected the former religious myths which gave meaning to life and we try to deny death, but we miss the social mechanisms and rituals which formerly made death easier to face. Studies of dying patients have shown that those with strong religious convictions and those who definitely do not believe in an after-life have least anxiety about death. It is the majority of people, with confused and contradictory beliefs, who are most likely to view their demise with alarm. Part of the fear of death is actually fear of the process of dying and patients need to be reassured on this score. It is now being recognised that the plight of patients who are terminally ill can represent a real failure in care and, in some places, a positive effort is being made to help staff to surmount their own anxieties in the interests of these neglected patients. As a result, the dying are being given privileges and choices which permit them to retain some semblance of human dignity and to share this final experience with their families.

Children in hospital

Children who enter hospital are in a special category. Their reaction will depend upon their age, the reason for admission, how far they have been prepared for it and, above all, the amount of continuing contact they can have with their parents. Since the 1959 Platt Report recommended unrestricted visiting of young children in hospital, a great deal has been learnt about the policies of different children's wards and the effect of the recommendations upon small patients and their families.

Once again, failures of communication between parents and staff have often been demonstrated, with some mothers being kept in the dark both regarding their children's illness and regarding their own entitlement to remain close at hand. It is often impossible to prepare a small child for what he will encounter in hospital, if only because many admissions are quite unexpected. The sudden separation from those who have hitherto been his loved protectors is potentially terrifying and should not be allowed to intensify his bewilderment and pain. A small proportion of children, who feel they have been totally abandoned, suffer severe, long-term effects from the experience. But the child's avoidable unhappiness should not be tolerated, whether or not its consequences are to be lasting.

However, the rigid organisation of some wards and hospitals does not easily adapt to the small child's individual needs. Nurses find considerable satisfaction in acting as mother substitutes and may not happily relinquish this opportunity, finding all sorts of reasons why it is inconvenient or unsuitable for the child's real mother to be present for long at a time. It may not be easy to accommodate outsiders to the ward and to find them a role which is not so insignificant as to be boring and ineffectual. The presence of parents, moreover, reveals all the staff's back-stage activities to the public gaze and this scrutiny may not be welcome, since nurses cannot perpetually put on an act of dramatic life-saving or suggest that they are constantly involved in vital clinical manoeuvres.

For their part, mothers may not appreciate the psychological value to the child of their being present and may find that the demands of the well members of their family must be given priority. Fathers may take the view that the hospital is doing everything necessary for the sick child and that the place of the wife and mother is at home. In addition, there are very real practical limits, in terms of available transport and money, upon the time which lower social class families can afford to spend with a sick child. In consequence, the actual amount of visiting which a child enjoys may depend on the distance of the hospital from his home.

A report of the Committee on Nursing has criticised the assumption underlying much research into the quality of nursing care, namely that the patient's health must show an improvement. In relation to several categories of patients who have already been mentioned in this chapter, the nursing element has been a component of care which is not necessarily directly related to cure. Where young children are concerned, it is clear that the provision of an environment which is not only physically comfortable but also emotionally satisfying and secure is very important in itself and should not require to be justified in terms of final results.

Mental illness and handicap

Turning to other areas where care is often inadequate, our society needs to face up to the realities of long term disabilities among the elderly, the young chronic sick, the mentally ill and the mentally subnormal. Many people in these categories still have to exist in ancient institutions, by no means suited to their current needs or in tune with the best modern concepts of treatment. After all, it is only recently that medicine has had so much success upon the technical side that doctors have felt free to contemplate the psychological implications of illness, so it is scarcely surprising if the public have not kept pace with these developments.

Erving Goffman gave a well-known account of the social life within some American mental hospitals, derived from his personal observation of patients and staff. He compared mental hospitals with other 'total institutions', places like prisons, military barracks and monasteries, in which the inmates have to live out all the aspects of their lives, and he conveyed a vivid impression of the indignities to which mental patients were subject. However, his memorable description failed to take due account of the underlying medical intention of most mental hospitals, namely their aim to restore sick people to normal functioning. The treatment of the mentally ill in Britain has improved markedly of late and a prolonged period of in-patient care is now exceptional. On balance it is to the advantage of people with a mental illness to be given the privileges of the sick role and to be cared for by doctors and nurses, in a place where diagnoses are carefully made and individual treatments prescribed and given.

The social atmosphere in which the treatment is provided and the attitudes of the staff are very important in the case of mental illness and it is in this field that the concept of the 'therapeutic community' has been most widely accepted and put into practice. As in the case of physical illness, it has proved difficult to demonstrate conclusively that the ward atmosphere actually contributes to cure and we are far from a final answer to chronic mental illnesses. But there can be little doubt that attitudes of optimism, tolerance and sympathy are more congenial and humane than the shameful and repressive regimes which, at some periods of our history, have characterised the care of the mentally ill.

Mental handicap

There is an important distinction to be made between mental illness and mental handicap or subnormality, since the situation of those who are permanently impaired is different from that of sick persons in whom cure, or at least some bettering of their condition, is anticipated. The reasons for any disablement are less important than the fact that it exists; the diagnosis matters less than the degree of impairment and disabled people generally are expected by society to behave as nearly as possible like normal citizens. Society, for its part, has a duty to help them to achieve their fullest possible potential. So much for the expectations and obligations relative to the impaired role.

However, some people are so crippled as to be unable to manage in the community and, in the worst instances, permanent care in an institution is necessary. Let us consider how this affects people who suffer from mental handicap, something quite unlike an illness, since recovery is never possible. The situation of the mentally handicapped represents a fascinating example of people who are uneasily poised between the society of the sick and the general community of the mentally and physically sound. Our culture has grown accustomed to dealing with physical illness. Over centuries acceptable rules and roles have been developed for all concerned and, within limits, our system of medicine has had a record of notable success in regard to diagnosis and cure. The mentally ill are in a marginal category, since the general public do not necessarily understand or accept the psychiatrists' definition of their condition as a sickness. But, on the whole, in Britain, they do receive proper care and attention. However, the mentally handicapped present a much more complicated problem for society and one which we are only now beginning to face up to and analyse properly. They consist of large numbers of people whose intelligence ranges from little below average (technically, an intelligence quotient of 70 per cent) to very severe grades of mental impairment and, at the lower levels, the mental deficiency is frequently associated with physical disabilities.

At the present time, in Britain, the population of hospitals for the mentally handicapped includes a high proportion of people (variously quoted as a half to two thirds) who might be able to live in the wider community, given certain pre-conditions. They do need the security of some kind of home where they can enjoy a degree of protective care and, secondly, they require a modicum of training so as to enable them to 'pass' in society. This is a very significant feature of their state; if they are to be accepted by the great mass of 'normal' people, they need a disguise, as otherwise they will be despised and rejected.

Robert Edgerton has used the phrase 'the cloak of competence' which admirably sums up the covering which the mentally subnormal require in order to conceal the nature of their infirmity from the unsympathetic public gaze. There is still a stigma attached to mental deficiency (and to mental illness too), a public reaction which is often painfully realised by the parents of a subnormal child.

Why is it, then, that so many individuals who are not sick are being confined in institutions which are modelled on hospitals for the physically ill? The answer lies largely in history for, originally, no distinction was drawn between those who were mentally impaired from birth and those who developed a mental illness in later life. They were all treated with mockery and neglect and often subjected to cruel restraints. In the late eighteenth century, certain humane and enlightened physicians, taking pity on the plight of these unfortunate people, instituted asylums where they could be protected and receive some kindly attention. The original idea of an asylum was a refuge or retreat from the harsh world outside.

As the reform movement was a medical initiative, these places were naturally regarded as hospitals and the staff who cared for the inmates were nurses. Later, as psychiatry developed as a medical speciality, doctors became aware of the difference between mental illness, which was potentially curable, and mental deficiency, which was a life-long condition. But the habit of caring for both groups in hospitals remained.

In the early years of this century an alarm was raised,

133

regarding what was then supposed to be the close relationship between crime and mental deficiency. Words like 'degeneracy' were freely used and people became obsessed with fears that if the mentally deficient were allowed to associate they would literally 'breed' all kinds of unpleasant social problems. In consequence, many people were put permanently away in institutions for reasons which had less to do with severe intellectual deficiencies than with the inadequacy of their own social environments and the prevailing attitudes of society at large. Although the fears of the eugenic alarmists have long ago been proved unfounded, it is still the case that many children have to be placed in large institutions for the mentally subnormal because there is insufficient support for them and their families in the community.

The social processes and changes in public and professional attitudes which have been briefly described are now well recognised. Just as medicine, in other spheres, has progressed to refinements of diagnoses and classification unknown in former times, so we are now in a position to classify people who are mentally deficient and to make accurate assessments of their particular needs, for education and training, for social support and, in the case of those with severe disabilities, for medical and nursing care.

Differences regarding optimum care

A recent government committee in Scotland (the Batchelor Report) made explicit recommendations which were based upon a rational assessment of the widely ranging needs of the mentally subnormal members of the population. The report made the controversial assertion that there is no such speciality as mental deficiency nursing. The subsequent Briggs Report (on nursing) has continued with this line of thought in its recommendations that all nurses in training should, in future, have experience of nursing the mentally deficient.

Such proposals are based on sound reasoning, but they encounter opposition at various levels. Nurses who have spent their lives in the care of the mentally deficient feel professionally threatened by the proposed changes and are sceptical of the capacity of their patients to survive in the competitive outside world. The public, democratically represented by local councillors, are reluctant to expend public funds on the reorganisation which such proposals would require since, in essence, it would mean removing large numbers of people right out of the category 'sick'. So long as people are 'sick' they are cared for in hospital and (in Britain) paid for by the central government. But, once this label is removed and they are no longer sick, the local community has to finance their care, and to balance their needs against those of all kinds of other unfortunates.

Once the topic of mental handicap is properly examined, it is clear that the handicapped need teachers, occupation therapists, speech therapists and a whole range of experts as well as nurses. Those whom it is proposed should in future live in the community, will need some people to care for them and to co-ordinate their care. Are such people necessarily nurses? In other words, do nurses have a caring monopoly or does their caring function derive from its medical connotations? A larger question would be to ask how far doctors should themselves concentrate on cure rather than care.

Thus we are left with conceptual and practical problems. The example on which we have spent some time, the social situation of the mentally subnormal, could easily be paralleled by that of the elderly, who represent a similar challenge to our society and to all the agents of health and welfare. Like the mentally handicapped, they occupy a lowly status and, for many reasons, they are without a powerful voice to press their own case.

The chronically disabled

Those who are chronically disabled, for whatever reason, are always liable to be given second place. Most of society consists of people who are active and striving to support themselves, their families and, incidentally, the national economy. But the impaired are a burden which the productive members of society have to bear. It is not without significance that the excellent and detailed recommendations which have repeatedly been made regarding the care of the elderly, the young chronically sick and the mentally handicapped have so far had depressingly little effect upon their actual circumstances. Many of these people continue to receive unsatisfactory care in outmoded institutions or sustain a precarious existence outside.

It may be that the attitudes of contemporary society are now altering in the direction of a greater consideration for the needs of those who cannot manage an independent existence, and that more money and research and staff will flow in that direction. However, until that happens, it seems as though many hospitals will continue to be their sole harbour and that nurses will continue the care which they alone have consistently provided hitherto. The new attempts to solve the problem of society's dependent members, with the prospect of hostels and day hospitals and half-way houses, are signs of an encouraging break with tradition. They are bound to present many challenges and problems to the nursing profession, since these are areas where the familiar, strict, hierarchical model is least appropriate but where the quality of the relationship between the nurse and her individual patient is of central importance.

Questions

1 What are the three main occupational groups working in hospital?

2 How is the nursing profession organised in hospital? Is there any single word or phrase which sums up this organisation?
3 How did the organisation of nursing come about and what are the reasons for its continuation today?
4 State some ways in which the organisation of the medical staff within hospital differs from that of the nursing staff.
5 Describe specific hospital situations in which the smooth co-operaton of nursing and medical staff is essential.
6 What is one of the major, unmet demands of patients in hospital? How do you think it could be satisfied?
7 Choose any one of these groups of patients and discuss the importance of good communications in relation to their needs—
   a Young children.
   b Maternity patients.
   c The dying.
8 Give some of the reasons why it is society finds it difficult to provide adequately for the needs of the chronically disabled. Illustrate your answer by reference to—
   a The elderly, or
   b The mentally handicapped.

Further reading

BARNES, ELIZABETH (1961) *People in Hospital*, Macmillan, London.

CARTWRIGHT, ANN (1964) *Human Relations and Hospital Care*, Reports of the Institute of Community Studies, Routledge & Kegan Paul, London.

ENGEL, GEORGE (1966) 'Grief and grieving', in *A Sociological Framework for Patient Care*, eds J. R. Folta and E. Deck, John Wiley, New York.

ENSING, E. C. (1966) *A New Look at Nursing*, Pitman Medical Publishing, London.

FRIEDSON, ELIOT (1963) ed., *The Hospital in Modern Society*, Free Press, New York.

GOFFMAN, ERVING (1968) *Asylums: Essays on the Social Situation of Mental Patients and other Inmates*, Penguin Books, Harmondsworth.

HINTON, JOHN (1967) *Dying*, Penguin Books, Harmondsworth.

HOUGHTON, H. (1968) 'Problems of hospital communication: an experimental study', in *Problems and Progress in Medical Care*, third series, Nuffield Provincial Hospitals Trust, Oxford University Press.

JONES, KATHLEEN (1955) *Lunacy, Law and Conscience 1744-1845*, Routledge & Kegan Paul, London.

MCGHEE, ANNE (1961) *The Patients' Attitude to Nursing Care*, E. & S. Livingstone, Edinburgh and London.

MENZIES, ISOBEL (1960) 'A case study in the functioning of social systems as a defence against anxiety: a report on a study of the nursing service of a general hospital', *Human Relations, 13*, 95-121.

MORRIS, PAULINE (1969) *Put Away: A Sociological Study of Institutions for the Mentally Retarded*, Routledge & Kegan Paul, London.

PATERSON, T. T. (1966) *Management Theory*, Business Publications, London.

PEARCE, EVELYN (1969) *Nurse and Patient: Human Relations in Nursing*, Faber & Faber, London.

REVANS, R. W. (1964) 'The morale and effectiveness of general hospitals', in *Problems and Progress in Medical Care*, 3rd series, Nuffield Provincial Hospitals Trust, Oxford University Press.

ROBERTSON, JAMES (1938) *Young Children in Hospital*, Tavistock Publications, London.

SKEET, MURIEL (1970) *Home from Hospital: A study of the home care needs of recently discharged hospital patients*, Dan Mason Nursing Research Committee, London.

SPENCER, J. A. (1967) *Management in Hospitals*, Faber & Faber, London.

STACEY, MARGARET, DEARDEN, ROSEMARY, PILL, ROISIN and ROBINSON, DAVID (1970) *Hospitals, Children and their Families*, Routledge & Kegan Paul, London.

TOWNSEND, PETER (1964) *The Last Refuge: A Survey of Residential Institutions and Homes for the Aged in England and Wales*, (abridged ed.) Routledge & Kegan Paul, London.

ZOLA, IRVING K. (1963) 'Problems of communication, diagnosis and patient care', *Journal of Medical Education, 38*, 829-38.

The Work of Nurses in Hospital Wards (1953), Nuffield Provincial Hospitals Trust.

Reports

The Reception and Welfare of In-Patients at Hospitals (1951), Report by Standing Advisory Committee, Department of Health for Scotland, HMSO, Edinburgh.

Welfare of Children in Hospital (1959), (Report of the Platt Committee), HMSO, London.

Human Relations in Obstetrics (1961), Standing Advisory Committee, Central Health Services Council, HMSO, London.

Visiting Patients in Hospital (1962), Report of a Committee, Scottish Home and Health Department, HMSO, Edinburgh.

Communication between doctors, nurses and patients: an aspect of human relations in the hospital service (1963) Ministry of Health, Report of a Joint Sub-Committee of the Central Health Services Council and the Ministry of Health, HMSO, London.

The Staffing of Mental Deficiency Hospitals (1970), Report of a Sub-Committee constituted jointly by the Standing Medical Advisory Committee and the Standing Nursing and Midwifery Advisory Committee (Chairman, I. R. C. Batchelor), HMSO, Edinburgh.

Report of the Committee on Nursing (1972) Cmnd 5115, Chairman, Asa Briggs, HMSO, London.

VI **The nurse in the community**

Implications for patients and nurses of separating branches of health service; community nursing in Britain to date; district nursing, differences in its content over time and between places; attachment schemes; health visitors' uncertain roles and new responsibilities; reasons for relative neglect of elderly in the community; basic conflict between concepts of prevention and cure; problems of disability and its treatment by society; increasing public demands for medical and nursing care; the midwives' dilemma; experiments in breaking hospital/community barriers; new divisions, between social work and nursing; future forms of community nursing in Britain; health centre organisation; nurse practitioners and medical assistants; nursing research; private nursing; nursing overseas; nursing in industry, opportunities and changes.

The nurse practising outside hospital, in the community, works in a very different social environment from that of her counterpart on the ward. Her relationships with patients, with doctors and with other nursing colleagues are likely to be considerably more varied and flexible than in an institutional setting, but the greater freedom and discretion which in general she experiences can be balanced by corresponding responsibilities and frustrations.

Nurses who work outside hospitals have been, until recently, in the great majority of cases, already trained. District nurses, midwives and health visitors have all completed the initial apprenticeship and have then acquired additional specialised qualifications, and they enjoy rewards of security and separate status denied to the student or pupil nurse. In future, the somewhat invidious distinctions between student and pupil nurse will probably disappear, to be replaced by an open career in nursing, starting from a common basis of certification. Upon this base, nurses may develop in the direction of their choice, whether their past basic training courses are towards hospital-centred practice or in the direction of community health. However, during their certificate training, all nurses will have been given some experience of community nursing.

Former health service organisation

Nurses in the community have hitherto been employed by a different branch of the health service, namely, the local health authorities, as opposed to the regional hospital boards which have run the hospitals. Added to this separation between hospital and home nursing went another significant division, since the doctors working in the community, the general practitioners, were administered by the third branch of the national health service, the executive councils. The historical and political reasons for this curious arrangement need not concern us here and, in fact, it is in course of disappearing with the re-organisation of the Health Service. Health boards are to be responsible for all the health needs of large areas of the country and will employ all the nursing and medical staff. The many disadvantages to patients, which result from the three-sided partition which has existed to date, have now been abundantly recognised. It was impossible to provide continuous care while such gaps between branches of the health service persisted.

The presence of three separate sections of the service had several significant effects on nursing practice. The divisions which have hitherto existed restricted community nurses to working in geographical areas, demarcated by local authority boundaries; they made any communication between hospital staff and staff employed by local authorities virtually non-existent; and they made it much more difficult to organise a working partnership between

141

doctors and nurses in the community for the common benefit of patients.

In this chapter we shall be looking at the various roles which nurses in the community have hitherto played and examining the possibilities for extensions and alterations in their functions, which the new health service re-organisation and the new proposals for nurse training now offer.

Away from the strict hierarchy of the hospital, nurses can often exercise a gratifying amount of autonomy. They are performing right in the front line of the organisation, a long way from the military style supervisors who officially command them. Although they belong to a similar hierarchy to that which defines the ranks and roles of senior nursing staff in hospitals, community nurses are nevertheless permitted, by the nature of their work, considerably more latitude and opportunities for personal initiative. For one thing, their superior officers are not physically present, as in the hospital; for another, since each nurse is working alone, she must often be prepared to make on-the-spot decisions about patients' care without the support of her peers or recourse to the precise instructions of her seniors.

District nursing

This is especially true in the case of home nurses, or district nurses, as they have usually been called in Britain. Since they were introduced over a hundred years ago they have built up a foundation of great public respect and trust. For many, the district nurse has epitomised the essential elements of her profession, hardworking, capable, compassionate and resourceful. She has provided patients and anxious relatives with the invaluable support of someone who is both professionaly competent and approachable, able to listen, advise and act.

Over the years the nature of the work done by district nurses has changed dramatically, in consequence of

142

advances in chemotherapy, changes in the age structure of the population and policies which encourage early discharge from hospital. Whereas formerly the district nurse was frequently involved in the home management of young people suffering from dangerous infections for which there was no specific cure, she is now largely concerned with patients with chronic illnesses or disabilities. Maintenance therapy, in the form of regular injections for diseases once rapidly fatal, like diabetes and pernicious anaemia, forms a significant part of her regular responsibilities. A great deal of her time is taken up with the needs of the sick and handicapped elderly, especially those who live alone or whose relatives are unable to cope with the exhausting and repetitive details of long-term personal care.

It is the district nurse who has been able to appreciate the importance of the family in illness and the devastating effects of the absence of supporting kin. Because she encounters so many poignant examples of loneliness and unhappiness and has personally to substitute for the attentions of absent relatives, she may be inclined to form a distorted picture of filial piety and wrongly conclude that most old people in Britain are deserted by their children.

She is the nurse who can realise the consequences for a family of having one of its members die slowly at home, from cancer or some other incurable condition; she observes the profound emotional and physical strains involved and provides vital, practical help for people who are near to breaking point.

Formerly, the district nurse might have been called in to help a patient through the crisis of lobar pneumonia, or in the course of meningitis, or to nurse a child slowly back to health after a severe and complicated infection. These were occasions fraught with drama and personal anguish, calculated to provoke the maximum responses of gratitude from the distraught members of the household. Today, she often continues to be associated with situations of real or potential danger, dealing with terminal illnesses and help-

ing the elderly to cope with unpleasant, disabling conditions. It is not surprising that she should be highly esteemed
nor that the thanks she receives should sometimes bear
scant relationship to the patient's recovery. Paradoxically,
she may be most effusively thanked by the relatives of
someone whom she has nursed through their last illness.
On the other hand, some of her elderly patients can be
very querulous and difficult to please. In some respects she
is heir to the affection and the difficulties which were once
the prerogative of the old-fashioned physician, in the days
when most illnesses were effectively beyond the range of
medical knowledge.

In country districts the home or district nurse holds a
special position, being well-known in the local community,
she can build up a fund of knowledge about all her potential
patients. Here, too, she is likely to be working in close
association with the local general practitioners serving the
same geographical area, and so she adds their need and
respect for her professional competence to that of her
patients.

Another feature of the nurse's work in remoter rural
areas, where distance makes the patient's contact with the
doctor difficult or infrequent, is that she is inevitably placed
on occasions in the position of having to make diagnostic
decisions and provide some medical advice. She will, for
example, sometimes be called upon for a first opinion by
her neighbours and she will then be obliged to estimate
the seriousness of their existing symptoms and whether it
is necessary to summon the distant doctor or recommend
attendance at his surgery. This informal arrangement is
likely to become much more frequent and deliberate in the
future. It is tied up closely with debates about the role
of medical assistants and we shall be returning to this
theme shortly.

District nurses have not always been happy about the
nature of the work they have had to undertake. In some
large towns nurses have considered that nearly a third of

their patients could just as well have been attended by an enrolled nurse, rather than by someone with their own superior qualifications. As in hospital, the work which any patient represents can be divided into tasks requiring more or less nursing skill and this poses problems of how to effect divisions which maximise nursing efficiency without sacrificing the patient's sense of security.

Careful comparative studies have shown that district nurses in towns spend more of their time on technical treatments than do their colleagues in country areas. Where hospitals are relatively inaccessible more sensible and extensive use is made of the home nurse's capacities and she is given more opportunity to provide basic nursing care and to supervise the patient's treatment personally. This is bound to be more satisfying than simply turning up on occasions to give injections or help old people in and out of bed. However, it is in the home that a nurse is best able to supply her patient with a multiplicity of attentions which all relate to his general comfort and well-being. It would be unfortunate if the total care of any one individual at home became fragmented as it often is in hospital. But there is little chance of this happening in the immediate future as it is highly unlikely that there will shortly be sufficient community nursing sisters, registered and certificated nurses, bath attendants, nursing aides and home helps to bring entire nursing teams to the bedsides of the majority of sick old people.

At the present time only a proportion of home nurses are restricted to performing one function, many of them being employed on the triple duties of home nursing, midwifery and health visiting. Alternatively, they may combine home nursing and midwifery. A combination of skills is commonest in country areas where it is both impractical and uneconomical to employ several types of nurse. In such places the nurse, in spite of varied duties, is likely to be less pressurised than in town and she may be able to provide for needs which are not met elsewhere, helping with minor illnesses in young people and giving advice on health in informal settings.

The country nurse in the community is less likely to be married than her urban counterpart, her district work often constitutes her main role and the house and car which accompany the job contribute to genuine professional and personal independence. Nurses who enter this branch of the profession often decide at an early age that they do not like the pressures of communal living and the constant presence of their seniors in hospital. They are anxious to embark upon practical work with patients in their own homes, finding the limitations imposed by ward routines both irksome and unsatisfying.

Although, theoretically, all patients should gain by having skilled nursing care available to them in their own homes, there is depressing evidence of the failure of the present system to bring this about on anything like a sufficient scale. A study which was made of the home care needs of patients recently discharged from hospital (Skeet, op. cit.) revealed a situation of appalling neglect, with many patients virtually abandoned once the hospital had finished with them. The health service had not developed any proper communication system between hospital staff and those nurses and doctors in the community who should be continuing treatment or ensuring a comfortable convalescence. Discharge occurred suddenly, without proper notice to relatives and medical and nursing staff and no prior assessment of the suitability of the home conditions was made by health visitors or social workers. Feeble old people were being unceremoniously decanted into cold empty houses, or sent back to die with relatives who were neither told how to cope nor supported by skilled assistance and finance.

Attachment schemes

In an attempt to provide patients in the community with better care and to allocate the skills of home nurses and doctors more equitably and effectively, a large number of attachment schemes have already been introduced and there is no doubt that this represents the future pattern of home care. Attachment is a formal arrangement whereby a nurse, midwife or health visitor has been responsible for providing services to patients on the lists of specified general practitioners. This has meant abandoning the former administrative allocation to geographical districts which so often produced unsatisfactory results for patients, nurses and doctors.

During the period when attachment was first being discussed, different ideas of its specific uses and advantages were mooted, largely dependent upon individual doctor's views of the proper roles for both parties and the extent to which they, as physicians, were prepared to envisage any change in their own usual modes of operating. Some doctors saw it as making their life easier, some nurses were equally determined not to be 'used' by the rival male profession, and some pessimistic commentators foretold that the patients would simply not stand for it.

There is now an impressive body of evidence on the effects of attaching existing district nurses to general practice. It has been tried out in many areas, sometimes with careful prior preparation and consultation, at other times as part of a sudden administrative process of 'unification'. One comprehensive review of attachment schemes discovered favourable reactions from both patients and doctors. Nurses did have much larger case loads but they generally welcomed the collaboration with doctors in the common care of patients about whom they were now much better informed. It also seemed as though nurses in this relationship with a doctor were likely to be entrusted with more responsible, supervisory duties instead of simply being ordered, anonymously, through the local authority, to administer routine treatments. Doctors who entered whole-heartedly into the schemes and got on well with the nurses concerned were of the impression that their own work was considerably lightened, allowing them time to extend their activities and improve their standards of practice.

However, there have been few attempts to measure the effects of attachment precisely, partly because it is extremely difficult to quantify the results for all the people concerned. A recent careful study in a large Scottish group practice set out with the declared aim of making the doctors more effective, by the optimum utilisation of district nurses who would deliberately be involved in some of the work previously performed solely by doctors. Measurements of the clinical activities of all the doctors and nurses were devised and the study was supplemented by regular dis-cussions with all concerned and by interviews with a sample of patients.

This was a more ambitious experimental scheme than most, since it went beyond the mere physical approxima-tion of nurses to doctors and introduced a redistribution of tasks and roles. Nurses went out on a variety of follow-up visits, they combined surgery duties with home nursing and they were engaged upon a considerable amount of work with young children who had infectious diseases or minor trauma. Following the addition of a state-enrolled nurse to the team, the district nurses specialised still more, covering a wider range of medical conditions on follow-up visits and helping to support neurotic and problem families. Patients frequently brought problems directly to the nurse, especially those relating to care following dis-charge from hospital. Occasionally, the nurse undertook fact-finding first visits if the doctor was unable to attend immediately and speed was essential. In fact, these district nurses were functioning as the future community clinical sisters will do.

The doctors, for their part, were able to concentrate more

148

on the consulting room and on their younger patients, confident that much routine home visiting and care was being competently discharged.

The great majority of patients sampled expressed themselves satisfied with the nurse's performance (88 per cent). A few parents had mild reservations and some adult patients had misunderstood the nurse's function and connections, not realising how close was her contact with their own doctor. However, some patients still maintained that, in future, they would prefer the doctor rather than the nurse to do the first follow-up visits after an illness. They definitely set the doctor's clinical competence at a higher level than that of the nurse and felt they were entitled to his superior skills, although they were prepared to acknowledge the nurse's abilities in the case of mild illness.

Health visiting

The role of the clinical nurse in the community is assured; long accepted by the public and welcomed by the doctor, she can look forward, in her metamorphosis from district nurse, to playing an increasingly important part in the community health care team. But her colleague the health visitor has often encountered problems of acceptance and recognition by both professionals and public. Like the familiar district nurse, she has, however, had a distinguished history and her unique contribution in the past was to the improvement in child welfare and the saving of infant lives.

Health visitors have been highly trained, being registered nurses with an additional year's theory and practice to fit them for providing health education and supervising the health of susceptible groups of people in the community. On average they have been recruited from families which are somewhat higher up the social scale than district nurses and possibly therefore more accustomed to a theoretical approach to problems. However this may be,

149

there has often been a certain coolness in relations between these two branches of nursing, one of which stresses the fundamental value of practical work with patients whilst the other sees disease prevention through education as a superior form of activity.

Changing roles

Until now, most of the work of health visitors has continued to relate to the needs of pre-school children, and they have frequently spent four times the amount of time upon paediatric care as on visits to the elderly. In spite of great changes in the health needs of the population, with old people predominating as patients in both general practice and hospital medicine, health visiting has continued to concentrate on routine visits to mothers with new babies. Whilst it is the case, as we have observed earlier, that many mothers are inadequately prepared for the experience of labour and are unsure about managing a small infant, it is highly doubtful whether the situation regarding health visitors' activities, which has existed hitherto, represents the correct use of skills or can be justified in terms of community need.

The health of the pre-school child in this country today is markedly better than it was a generation ago. Standards of hygiene and nutrition have improved, the deficiency diseases of the past have disappeared, and immunisation and chemotherapy have contributed to the defeat of many previously dangerous infections. Moreover, the health service provides free primary care on demand to all young children and most mothers are well-accustomed to visiting or calling their doctors if a child is unwell. There are important exceptions to the sensible utilisation of child care services, but the majority of families are sufficiently motivated and well-informed.

The elderly sector of the population, however, not only experiences more ill health and disability but is less likely to make full use of medical services. Why, then, do health visitors persist in visiting babies?

There are a number of reasons for this anomalous situation. Since the early days of public health, society has acknowledged its responsibility for the care of its youngest members and the provision of special clinics for small infants was introduced long before the inauguration of a free health service for the population as a whole. In other words, there is a long history of investment in the young who, it is hoped, will presently grow up to be useful, active members of society. Society's responsibility to the elderly is of a different nature, being more in the nature of a payment for past service than an investment in future potential. As we remarked in the previous chapter, in any society which is orientated towards production and achievement, those who can no longer work and strive unfortunately tend to become second-class citizens. Their claim to public attention requires to be loudly and persistently pressed by others and their needs can easily be neglected if the health and welfare services are badly organised or if alternative demands upon resources are more strongly advocated.

Relative neglect of the elderly

In fact, old people are among the main victims of the structure and methods of working which have characterised the existing health service. Although everyone is on the list of a general practitioner, our system of primary health care depends upon self referral. That is to say, a person has to decide for himself that he is sick enough to need medical help. Once he or she attends the doctor and is officially labelled as being sick, all the resources of modern medicine may, theoretically, be brought to bear upon their condition.

But, in the case of old people, their sickness is often inextricably tied up with their social circumstances and the mental and physical weakness which are part of growing old may reduce their inclination or capacity to seek help. Added to this is their tendency to accept some degree of disability with cheerful resignation. Meanwhile, there are trained people around who might help and advise them or who might bring a doctor to attend them.

But this is where the administrative problem begins to obtrude, because health visitors have, until lately, been in the employment of local authorities who know neither the names nor the whereabouts of the old people in an area and who have no 'right' to visit them. The doctor is the one person given privileged access by society to the homes and bodies of the sick. But local authority employees are not in this privileged category, even if they are part of the local health department. Since their function is preventive and not curative, they are without personal authority to invade the homes of private citizens.

In the case of small children the matter is different because, in the first place, their identities and addresses are easily obtainable, since their births have just been officially registered and, second, because society has come to accept the well-intentioned home visits of a nurse from the health department. It is easier for people generally, whether they are parents, teachers or nurses, to dictate what happens to small, dependent members of society, than to presume to advise other adults upon the conduct of their lives.

There are, fortunately, ways out of this dilemma, one of the most obvious being to have health visitors working in conjunction with doctors, thereby rendering their own activities at once more acceptable, more extensive and more medically orientated. Since the doctor has a list of everyone in his practice, young and old, and since he is regarded nowadays as a legitimate health promoter as well as a healer, the health visitor in this situation can gain access to more homes through her symbolic and actual association with him.

Health visitors' special skills

Not only can this connection help the health visitor to uncover the hidden health needs of elderly people, it can also modify her image in the eyes of the rest of the public. Whereas the old style district nurse has derived great advantages from her positive role in helping the sick, so that she is the recipient of affectionate regard, the health visitor's image is associated with that of a teacher, a somewhat more distant, authoritative figure liable to point out errors and disapprove of social lapses. Health visitors themselves do not like to be remembered as 'public health nurses', but this discarded epithet did serve to remind people of their nursing background. The health visitor's background and specialised training is often not properly appreciated by her potential clients. Some doctors are disgracefully vague regarding the health visitor's special skills and, where they do partly understand her qualifications, may consider that her prior practical training is being wasted upon purely educative tasks. They may not realise her potential as regards assessment and monitoring functions in the community.

Combined duties

Other countries do not necessarily make the division between health visiting and home nursing which we take for granted but have a category of community nurses to perform both functions. As has been remarked earlier, in many parts of Britain nurses do perform combined duties and the proposed new community health sisters may undertake a certain amount of what is rather ambiguously termed 'nursing support'.

There are many opportunities for health education which a nurse who enters a home is ideally placed to utilise. At a time of illness people are particularly receptive to lessons which are clearly relevant to their current circumstances

153

and both patients and their relatives are motivated to pay special attention. The nurse can pass on vital instructions in nursing techniques which will make the family more capable of looking after a patient themselves. The observation of her activities is likely, incidentally, to affect watching children, who will absorb some of these lessons and act them out at play.

However, nurses who have tried to carry out both roles have often reported that the burden of home nursing seems to reduce the time they manage to spend on the health education or health visiting side of their work. Partly this is a consequence of overall shortages, since the claims of the sick must inevitably take precedence over the well. In some of the largest group practices and in new health centres, resources may permit the employment of a wide range of health care specialists, whereas, when the population is scanty and scattered, people are obliged to double up and to do jobs which might be delegated elsewhere.

To a large extent, the situation in the community parallels that in hospitals, which can be ranked according to the number and kinds of specialised professionals they employ. The professorial departments of metropolitan teaching hospitals have at their disposal medical specialists, nurses, auxiliaries and attendants of every grade and degree, whereas isolated general hospitals or institutions for the chronically sick and impaired must make do with fewer, less clever doctors and depend upon many untrained nurses.

Prevention versus cure

However, the difficulties attendant upon practitioners of preventive medicine, whether they are community physicians or health visitors, are not entirely explicable in organisational or resource terms. The fundamental problem relates to the public's view of health and disease, their definition of which categories of people require medical care and the extent to which they are prepared to admit the activities of doctors and nurses into the lives of those who do not conceive of themselves as being sick.

Doctors are used to the concept of 'at risk' groups in the community, meaning by this term people whose circumstances or experiences predispose them to the development of ill health. It is by now widely accepted that it is desirable to protect vulnerable small children from certain diseases through immunisation. The scientific basis for this technical procedure is probably understood by very few people, but it is taken on trust, as a quasi-magical protective device. Parents, as a rule, feel very solicitous for their children's welfare and are open to professional suggestions for ensuring their optimum health. It is, however, much more difficult to convince middle-aged or elderly adults who feel reasonably fit that they need medical surveillance or that their inclusion in a statistical category permits preventive medicine specialists, of one sort or another, to interfere with them. Doctors and nurses may feel fairly convinced of the likelihood of discovering symptoms of physical or mental ill health among the very old or among certain groups of middle-aged people. But the public's perceptions of what constitutes sickness may not have caught up with the views of the most enlightened practitioners. In consequence, there are barriers to the institution of widespread screening programmes which relate to community attitudes as well as to community resources.

At the same time, however, the idea is growing that people have a 'right to health'. This is almost entirely a concern of the fortunate inhabitants of countries in the Western world which have a highly developed economy and a high standard of living. Elsewhere in the world, where many dangerous diseases are still rampant, modern medicine is still mainly seen as an aid to mere survival, although traditional medical systems have their prophylactic aspect. Indeed, even in the Western world, the belief that 'health' is a normal condition of being which doctors and nurses should actively encourage and maintain, is largely the assumption of the richer members of society. The old and the poor can scarcely presume to such expectations and are more inclined to accept as inevitable some degree of disability or discomfort. It could half seriously be suggested that proper attention to the needs of old people might have to wait acceptance of the view that 'old' and 'sick' are near synonymous terms.

The disabled in society

The question of how to provide adequate medical care and counsel for the underprivileged members of our own society, those who are permanently disabled and lack a powerful voice, is one which transcends the matter of practice organisation and health service administration. It is rooted in the attitudes of society towards people who are unproductive and, consequently considered relatively unimportant. Though we have developed clear views as to how to treat the sick, granting them privileges of dependence and absolving them temporarily from effort in the interests of rapid return to full function, we expect the disabled to behave as much as possible like normal people and not to parade impairments about which little can effectively be done. Although doctors may realise that the division between sickness and impairment is very difficult to draw in practice, and that minor complaints can be prevented, by prompt attention, from developing into permanent disabilities, this sophisticated medical viewpoint is not common amongst laymen.

Even doctors and nurses find it hard to balance the advantages of early reporting of symptoms by patients against the extra work which they constantly fear may result from 'unnecessary' consultations. Their own allegiance to the ideal of prevention rather than cure is by no means wholehearted It has, of course, repeatedly been

demonstrated that the provision of extra medical facilities
and diagnostic clinics multiplies rather than diminishes the
work of health professionals. A case in point is the experience of those practices which have adopted nurse attachments, where the nurses' work load increases and the
doctor soon finds outlets for the time which he supposedly
saves.

Increasing demand for medical care

The demand for medical care in a modern state seems
to be literally inexhaustible and public expectations are
bound to increase at a rate which constantly outstrips the
provision of care. When there is the possibility of treatment, people's tolerance of minor symptoms is reduced and
they begin to expect medication for all sorts of unpleasant
sensations and experiences. For example, the availability
of tranquillisers encourages reliance upon drugs which
modify the harsh impact of reality and dull the pain of
loss.

Nurses who work in the community are subject to the
pressures of changing public demand in a way which their
colleagues in hospital can seldom appreciate, shielded as
they are by the fixed apparatus of beds and strict admission
policies. The hospital has managed to remain remarkably
isolated from the community it serves, secure in its position
as the repository of ultimate skills and transcendent
medical mysteries. The isolation of hospitals from the community has stemmed from history and has been perpetuated
by administrative convenience. But now there are welcome
indications that this traditional exclusiveness is in process
of erosion.

The midwives' dilemma

For example, as was mentioned in the previous chapter,
our country has developed the policy of encouraging the

great majority of mothers to have their babies in hospital. This has had, however, the incidental effect of depriving many district midwives of the satisfaction of exercising their central skills. Some hospitals have encouraged community midwives to enter their hallowed precincts for the purpose of attending in labour those patients whose pregnancy they have already supervised. Community midwives who miss out entirely on confinements naturally feel cheated of a vital part in the drama of birth. Engaged only in preparatory and residual rituals, they are unnaturally deprived of performing their rightful role.

Indeed, the midwife today does experience very considerable role confusion. Formerly she had a unique position among nurses, being statutorily empowered to carry out deliveries herself, and only being required to call in a doctor if an exceptional case was presenting complications. Most of her work was outside hospital, in the patients' own homes, and she was able to tend women right through their pregnancy, labour and puerperium. Because of the move towards hospital confinement, the majority of midwives now work within the ward structure, where they encounter the disciplines characteristic of the nursing profession generally and where the medical staff are likely to be constantly at hand. As an article by Jean Walker has pointed out, the hospital midwife may feel that there is little to distinguish her from a maternity nurse, and that she has lost some of her traditional and distinctive autonomy. Even in the community, if she is working alongside a GP, the amount of personal responsibility she is given is liable to vary quite arbitrarily, depending on the doctor's own zeal for ante-natal care and occasional obstetrics. She can, of course, perform a valuable educational function during pregnancy, but the important lessons she has to give will be more effective if she can follow them through with the patient, during the experiences of childbirth and early childrearing.

Joining hospital and community care

To retain the services of domiciliary midwives in circumstances when their skills are least required and utilised is damaging to their self-image and status and can also affect the patient's emotional security, since a mother can relate more easily and closely to someone who has steered her through the actual birth process and its immediate sequel. Some hospitals have begun a counter movement, outwards from the hospital into the community, by arranging that follow-up visits to patients delivered in hospital should be undertaken, at least for ten days, by the hospital midwife who attended the mother and baby. The object of this innovation is not merely the provision of comforting continuity of care, though the mothers do appreciate this. It can also mean earlier discharge and, consequently, a more rapid turnover in the wards. A further important advantage of this arrangement stems from the fact that the care of the new-born infant has now become a distinct nursing and medical speciality and it is often in the best interests of the baby that it should be followed up by someone in a position to know its detailed neo-natal history and special needs. The midwife needs to appreciate the profound effect which social and cultural factors have upon the health and development of very young children. Although it is likely that most midwives will be hospital-based in future, a movement into the community will preserve a sense of the importance of the infant's social setting.

Related to the outward-looking development in the field of midwifery has been the experiment of attaching district nurses to the surgical departments of general hospitals in order to follow patients after their discharge and continue at home treatments which would otherwise have required a longer stay in an expensive hospital bed. In other cases, home nurses or health visitors have combined association with particular general practices along with attendance in

159

hospital, or they have acted as a link between a hospital speciality, such as geriatrics or paediatrics, and the services in the community. These eminently sensible arrangements have resulted in increased patient satisfaction, saving of hospital beds, better communication with doctors and a more satisfying job for the nurses concerned. In view of the desperate gaps in patient care which have hitherto resulted from the hospitals' separation from the community, further experiments designed to break down the communication barriers should certainly be encouraged, whatever their disadvantages to the tidy administrative mind.

These developments bear a resemblance to certain new medical situations, where general practitioners are taking a part in the hospital care of their own patients and even, at times, having a part-time hospital appointment and extending their province to care for in-patients not on their own practice lists. This fulfils an appreciable professional demand for more participation in the scene 'where the action is'. In the case of doctors, there are certain difficulties and drawbacks, relating to their dubious status in this situation as quasi-consultants. These criticisms should not apply to nurses and midwives, however, whose training ought already to fit them for continuing treatments and supervision begun in hospital. Other nurses, participating in special studies of patients, should certainly have the opportunity of crossing traditional boundaries.

There is no point in pretending, however, that such innovations are easy or likely to meet with ready acceptance from all concerned. The nursing profession, like other occupations, has developed traditional job demarcations, role prescriptions and expectations, and its component subdivisions often cherish those very differences which contribute to a sense of identity and importance. Thus, health visitors may not relish the invasion of their territory by midwives-in-training and surgical ward nurses may look askance at the outsiders who briefly penetrate their exclusive preserves. It has even sometimes been the case that those who were officially termed 'district' nurses have been specifically warned against exploitation in the form of sessions in the GP's surgery. Health visitors, in particular, resent any suggestion of a return to those practical tasks which their training has entitled them to relinquish and will stress the counselling, assessment and supervisory aspects of their calling.

Divisions between social work and nursing

But, if different members of the same profession are sensitive regarding the correct deployment of their respective skills, they are even more suspicious of the imagined threat which is posed by total outsiders, in the shape of social workers. Since it is health visitors and social workers who have most in common, they are probably the nurses who are most preoccupied at the moment about the division of disputed territory.

Until recently, the health visitor employed by the health department of a local authority might anticipate that her work would include helping families who had social problems, at least to the extent of advising them where to go for help. Her training had included lectures and practical projects in sociology and she had learned about the organisation of the health and welfare services. She might also expect to be in contact with the mentally disordered and people who were abnormally disabled for any reason. However, the expansion of social work has meant a corresponding reduction in areas with which health visiting was formerly charged. The uncertainty regarding the future which many health visitors feel is partly a consequence of their persistent emphasis upon a teaching role, which comes rather closer to the advice giving and directional role of their non-medical contemporaries in social work than to the home nursing which their other community colleagues still practice. Health visitors have occasionally feared that, since they have emphasised teaching and

161

health education as their main function, they might logically be associated with education departments, if they were
to continue to be employed by local authorities. In the final
analysis, however, their nursing role has taken precedence
over their teaching role, and their relationship with the
health services has meant that they will be part of the
Area Health Board organisation which integrates home
and hospital services.

This is not the place to discuss in detail the problems
of social workers today in respect to their own role
definitions, nor to compare their ideal self-image with the
actual jobs which client pressures force upon them. It
should be sufficient to say that the most articulate spokes-
men of social workers usually feel that their function goes
beyond that of being mere signposts to welfare benefits and
includes a therapeutic aspect in the efforts to help families
in trouble to deal personally with their problems and
difficulties.

As has been said repeatedly in this book, the division
between social and medical problems is seldom easy to
draw, and the degree to which doctors will implicate themselves in their patients' social situations is largely a matter
of personal and professional preference. However, regard-
less of individual doctors' attitudes towards the psychological or social side of their patients' complaints, the
fact remains that a great many people today do go to their
doctors for help and advice with matters which are not
purely medical. There are many reasons for this, to do
with the relative decline in reliance on religious advisers
and the shortage of convenient kin to supply people with
homely counsel. From the point of view of the doctor to
whom various problems are brought, these people in need
often represent clients whom he is simply not qualified to
serve, never having been trained to find a way through the
welfare jungle or taught to supply the special brand of
support which they may require.

It is not surprising, therefore, that the most advanced

and adventurous group practices and health centres should hope for the attachment of social workers and perceive advantages in a closer association with social work colleagues comparable to those deriving from nurse attachments.

In the circumstances, it is somewhat unfortunate that social workers, determined upon their establishment as a distinct profession, should recently have removed themselves decisively from the administrative neighbourhood of the rival medical camp. Legislation has set up social work departments in local authorities almost at the same time as the health functions of local authorities were being entirely removed and transferred to Regional and Area Health Boards

Social workers have for long bewailed their inferior status in relation to medicine and resented the uninformed and patronising manner towards them of doctors who have misunderstood and misused their capacities. They are now struggling to set up their own exclusive hierarchical structures and teams and are in process of distributing the multiple community duties for which they are responsible. There is, therefore, little possibility that doctors can automatically expect social workers to operate for them directly or that social workers will helpfully range the GP's practices to select and settle 'social problems'.

But, if the doctor can never hope to possess and command the social worker, it should be feasible to bring about useful co-operation on the basis of mutual consultation. Indeed there are a number of instances where doctors in a group practice, already well staffed with several grades of nurses, have arranged regular case conferences with social workers in the same neighbourhood. Provided that the doctor does not 'pull rank' with his social work colleagues and provided there is a free exchange of information, these arrangements seem to facilitate purposeful decisions and bring co-ordinated care to the service of families in trouble. As in the case of closer contact between doctors and nurses, the co-operation across professional boundaries can prove mutually beneficial and educative.

The future of community nursing

The future pattern of community health care in this country will undoubtedly be based upon health centres and group practices. General practice has experienced an amazing renaissance in Britain and doctors all over the country have been experimenting with ways of delivering comprehensive care to families who are in all kinds of difficult circumstances. Already many different forms of organisation are being tried out, utilising a multiplicity of doctors, nurses, midwives, aides, attendants, receptionists and secretarial staff and hopefully incorporating at the same time active connections with social work department personnel. The team is rapidly replacing the single-handed, personal physician and specialisation is the order of the day.

If the Briggs recommendations for nurse training are implemented, the future structure of community nursing will reflect the needs of the vast majority of the population who live outside hospitals and who must be supplied with preventive as well as clinical services. There will be a broad division, on the nursing front, into those who supply skilled nursing care and treatment for patients at home or in medical premises of one sort or another, and those whose joint responsibility is towards the well community and the chronically disabled. The two types of nurse will be called, respectively, family clinical sisters and family health sisters, thus drawing attention to a fundamental distinction in their social roles and allegiance. Thus, whereas the clinical sisters will be supporters of the sick and constantly engaged in active efforts to reverse the sick role of their patients, the health sisters will always emphasise normality, trying to keep people well by giving sound advice and, where this is impossible because someone is quite clearly disabled, stressing those measures which will enable the handicapped to live as 'normal' a life as possible. The new division in community nursing precisely reflects the differing attitudes of society towards the sick and the disabled to which we have repeatedly made reference in this book. Since it has the joint attractions of sociological sense and logicality it is to be hoped that this new concept of community nursing can be introduced in practice. There can, however, be no disguising the difficulties which may arise over what necessitates a blurring in the former distinctions between the roles of district nurse and health visitor. From one point of view, the proposed new system will simply be generalising on the situation which has often existed in practice where the roles of health educator and nurse have combined. But it may occasionally prove hard to separate 'clinical nursing' from 'nursing support' and it would be most unfortunate if demarcation disputes were to mar the improvements in patient care which are anticipated under the new arrangements.

However these minor differences are resolved, and the solution undoubtedly lies in establishing new images and then providing the training to promote them, community nurses will be a prominent feature of the future health service.

Health centre teams

It is impossible to predict the commonest form which the new organisation of community medical care will take. But it is clear, as we have suggested earlier, that they are liable to resemble hospital out-patient departments more than traditional family doctors' surgeries. Although the word 'team' is much in vogue its implications remain to be worked out. For example, a team implies a leader. But, as we have seen, doctors and nurses have different professional notions of leadership and hierarchies. For

165

example, will all the members of a health centre team constitute a semi-autonomous unit? It seems much more probable that nurses will be managed directly by nursing officers in their own speciality. After a century of freedom fighting, the nursing profession could not conceivably submit to working in small medical oligarchies. Then as far as the doctors are concerned, will they all be equal or will some be 'more equal' than others? Will a medical, or non-medical administrator be necessary or will some form of local democracy or government by committee be preferred? Where there are several grades and types of nursing staff there will certainly be an official leader of the nursing team. In view of the training in management which senior nursing officers now receive, would not a nursing officer be suitable for overall administration? These are only a few of the questions relating to the internal organisation of health centres, the answers to which will have an enormous influence on their effective operation. Clearly, there is room for great variation and much is bound to depend on factors such as size, siting and the numbers and types of staff.

There is a real danger, if health centre organisation becomes very large, that patients' primary needs for accessible and easily available care may be overlooked. Such a centre or polyclinic may be considerably further from the patient's home than the former, convenient GP's surgery. Once at the centre the patient may find it consists of a confusing maze of separate stations, each staffed by unknown personnel. In primary care 'biggest' does not necessarily mean 'best'.

Medical assistants and nurse practitioners

In other parts of the world, shortage of doctors to work in primary medical care has combined with nurses' dissatisfaction with their traditional roles to produce many variants on the patterns to which we are accustomed. There are moves towards increased specialisation of nursing in somes places and towards the production of new varieties of medical assistant, part doctor part nurse, in others.

Nurse practitioners in the USA and Canada have received additional training to fit them for expanded roles and increased responsibilities in the delivery of primary medical care. They are intended to work in collaboration with family doctors and to assume responsibilities which include assessment of a patient's or a family's health problems, the health education of individuals and families, monitoring of patients with chronic conditions, pre- and post-natal supervision of mothers and assessment of the development of young children and adolescents. This wide range of functions spans those which we have been accustomed to divide between district nurses, health visitors and community midwives. Once the Canadian nurse practitioner is trained, for example, she may operate in a number of different settings and the nature of her work will vary with the circumstances. Thus she may be a member of a large health care team in an urban area; in some outposts, she may effectively act as a substitute physician, discharging diagnostic and therapeutic responsibilities which are normally those of a doctor; in other places she may be a 'physician associate', closely corresponding to our idea of a family clinical sister attached to a doctor's practice.

The USA, the world's most affluent country, has lately been experiencing a crisis in primary health care. The urban ghettoes and the poor country areas are unpopular places for doctors to practise in, since the impoverished inhabitants of both are unable to pay high medical fees. At the same time many medical orderlies discharged from the American armed forces have been in search of suitable employment and eager to undertake sufficient further training to become medical assistants. They now form a significant para-medical group who, in some areas, constitute a threat to the doctors' former autonomy. Their attitude towards nurses is interesting. The medical assistants are all men and they resent the fact that the women of the long-established nursing profession are being accorded higher status, higher salaries and better career prospects.

Although medical assistants are new to America, Russia has a long tradition of employing 'feldschers'. Originally barber surgeons to the Tsar's armies, their present-day counterparts perform a wide variety of tasks in the community. As in other parts of the world, their responsibilities vary; in country areas they are able to take more independent decisions and are less subject to direction, whereas in towns their role as 'assistant' doctors is emphasised and less 'substitution' occurs.

As was mentioned in a previous chapter, the ex-colonial empire now has many different kinds of medical assistants, with varying lengths of training. Like the feldschers and the American medical assistants, they too have military origins, having been first introduced as part of the army-style colonial medical services.

In China, the 'barefoot doctors' are very young school-leavers who are trained in only a few basic elements of health care but who are nevertheless able to supply some medical attention for people who would otherwise be totally bereft.

Countries which already have a long tradition of nursing training are inclined to develop new and more specialised types of nurses rather than favouring the introduction of a separate group of medical assistants to cope with new needs. However, even highly developed countries face the insoluble equation of boundless demands and limited resources. Everywhere scarce skills have to be economically deployed in a situation where demand outstrips supply. It is nowhere practicable to think in terms of doctors working single-handed; since there are always many patients to every doctor, the question becomes one of marshalling all the available diagnostic, assessment and caring skills to the best advantage of the community.

Nursing research

Some nurses may elect to specialise in the study of their own performance and engage in research. The material for their consideration is certainly wide and complex, covering all the fields with which this book has dealt and demanding special training and mental discipline. Several places in Britain are actively encouraging nursing research, which is seen as not simply the preoccupation of a few gifted individuals but as a prerequisite for the proper self-knowledge of the entire profession.

Nursing overseas

Some nurses trained in Britain are bound to go abroad. They may practice in developing countries, where they are likely to be given a great deal of clinical and management responsibility and be required to exercise initiative and imagination. Faced with cultures very different from their own they can benefit enormously by studying the background from which their patients come and trying to discover all that is known regarding local beliefs about health and sickness, diet, and traditional ways of rearing children. With an appreciation of sociology, supplemented by anthropological information, the nurse in a foreign country may avoid the worst blunders of the outsider and is much more likely to be successful in health education.

Private nursing

Other nurses, who stay in Britain, may opt for the relatively independent position of private nursing. They may elect to register with an agency and move around from one job and setting to another. There is sometimes a tendency to regard the private operator as a hardened self-seeker and to imply that her standards and welfare are bound to suffer from lack of stimulating and supportive contact with others in her profession. But this attitude may partly stem from the fact that the nursing norm is bureaucratic, and the nurse who chooses private enterprise need trade neither efficiency nor morality in the process.

Nursing in industry

The nurse in industry is in a separate but interesting situation, particularly if the firm which employs her is large and health-conscious. Here, although she will be part of a big organisation, it will be quite unlike a hospital, because everyone is well most of the time, and she may be working closely with the factory doctor, but without senior nurses' directions.

Changing responsibilities

The nursing scene in Britain today is one of great change and promise, offering a vast range of experiences, from work in the most specialised intensive care units or in large, urban health centres to the responsibilities of community nursing in a remote country setting. Nurses can shortly expect modifications in their roles and may be required to expand their functions in ways and directions which their predecessors could never have imagined. With the re-organisation of the health service and the changes in nurse training, the opportunities for co-operation between the nursing and medical profession are greatly expanded. In these changing times and shifting circumstances, it is always wise to remember that any health service is designed for patients and that all those who serve should try to put the patient's welfare first.

Questions

1 Describe some of the ways in which divisions within the

Health Service have interfered with the complete nursing care of patients.

2 What are the difficulties and rewards of district nursing? How may the work vary between town and country?
3 What does the term 'triple duties' mean to you?
4 How may an 'attachment scheme' work in general practice, as far as the nurse is concerned?
5 How has it come about that health visiting hitherto has mainly involved families with young children?
6 Give some reasons for the comparative neglect of the elderly in our society.
7 List some of the advantages and disadvantages of separating health education from practical nursing.
8 Describe some of the personnel whom other countries have trained to supplement their health services.
9 What will probably be the future types of community nurse in Britain and what will be their respective responsibilities?

Further reading

CARSTAIRS, VERA (1966) *Home Nursing in Scotland*, Scottish Health Services Studies, 2, Scottish Home and Health Department.

GOFFMAN, ERVING (1968) *Stigma: Notes on the Management of Spoiled Identity*, Penguin Books, Harmondsworth.

HOCKEY, LISBETH (1968) *Care in the Balance*, Queens Institute of District Nursing, Severs, Cambridge.

HOCKEY, LISBETH (1970) 'District nursing sister attached to hospital surgical department', in *The New General Practice II*, British Medical Association, BMA House, London.

JEFFREYS, MARGOT (1965) *An anatomy of social welfare services*, Ch. VI, 'The health visiting service', and Ch. VII, 'The district nurse and midwifery service', Michael Joseph, London.

KING, MAURICE (1966) ed., *Medical Care in Developing Countries*, Oxford University Press, London.

MACGREGOR, S. W., HEASMAN, M. A. and KUENSSBERG, E. V. (1971) *The evaluation of a direct nursing attachment in a North Edinburgh practice*, Scottish Health Services Studies, 18, Scottish Home and Health Department.

SKEET, MURIEL (1970) *Home from Hospital: A study of the*

home care needs of recently discharged hospital patients, Dan Mason Nursing Research Committee.

STOCKS, MARY (1960) *A Hundred Years of District Nursing*, Allen & Unwin, London.

WALKER, JEAN (1972) 'The changing role of the midwife', *International Journal of Nursing Studies, 9*, 85-94.

YOUNG, WILLIAM C. (1971) 'A work study of nursing staff in a Health Department', *Health Bulletin, 29*, 154-61.

The New General Practice II (1970), articles published in the *British Medical Journal.*

World Health, The Magazine of the World Health Organization (1972) 'Medical assistants—what's in a name?'

Reports

Attachment of Nursing Services in General Practice (1970), Report of a Joint Working Party on Group Attachment, Educare, Hemel Hempstead.

Living with Handicap (1970), Report of a Working Party on Children with Special Needs, National Bureau for Co-operation in Child Care, London.